T0263442

Vascular Ultrasound

Guest Editors

DEBORAH RUBENS, MD
EDWARD G. GRANT, MD

ULTRASOUND CLINICS

www.ultrasound.theclinics.com

Consulting Editor
VIKRAM S. DOGRA, MD

October 2011 • Volume 6 • Number 4

SAUNDERS an imprint of ELSEVIER, Inc.

W.B. SAUNDERS COMPANY
A Division of Elsevier Inc.

1600 John F. Kennedy Boulevard • Suite 1800 • Philadelphia, Pennsylvania 19103-2899

http://www.theclinics.com

ULTRASOUND CLINICS Volume 6, Number 4
October 2011 ISSN 1556-858X, ISBN-13: 978-1-4557-1160-4

Editor: Barton Dudlick
Developmental Editor: Donald Mumford

© **2011 Elsevier Inc. All rights reserved.**

This journal and the individual contributions contained in it are protected under copyright by Elsevier, and the following terms and conditions apply to their use:

Photocopying
Single photocopies of single articles may be made for personal use as allowed by national copyright laws. Permission of the Publisher and payment of a fee is required for all other photocopying, including multiple or systematic copying, copying for advertising or promotional purposes, resale, and all forms of document delivery. Special rates are available for educational institutions that wish to make photocopies for non-profit educational classroom use. For information on how to seek permission visit www.elsevier.com/permissions or call: (+44) 1865 843830 (UK)/(+1) 215 239 3804 (USA).

Derivative Works
Subscribers may reproduce tables of contents or prepare lists of articles including abstracts for internal circulation within their institutions. Permission of the Publisher is required for resale or distribution outside the institution. Permission of the Publisher is required for all other derivative works, including compilations and translations (please consult www.elsevier.com/permissions).

Electronic Storage or Usage
Permission of the Publisher is required to store or use electronically any material contained in this journal, including any article or part of an article (please consult www.elsevier.com/permissions). Except as outlined above, no part of this publication may be reproduced, stored in a retrieval system or transmitted in any form or by any means, electronic, mechanical, photocopying, recording or otherwise, without prior written permission of the Publisher.

Notice
No responsibility is assumed by the Publisher for any injury and/or damage to persons or property as a matter of products liability, negligence or otherwise, or from any use or operation of any methods, products, instructions or ideas contained in the material herein. Because of rapid advances in the medical sciences, in particular, independent verification of diagnoses and drug dosages should be made.

Although all advertising material is expected to conform to ethical (medical) standards, inclusion in this publication does not constitute a guarantee or endorsement of the quality or value of such product or of the claims made of it by its manufacturer.

Ultrasound Clinics (ISSN 1556-858X) is published quarterly by W.B. Saunders, 360 Park Avenue South, New York, NY 10010-1710. Months of publication are January, April, July, and October. Business and editorial offices: 1600 John F. Kennedy Boulevard, Suite 1800, Philadelphia, Pennsylvania 19103-2899. Accounting and circulation offices: 6277 Sea Harbor Drive, Orlando, FL 32887-4800. Periodicals postage paid at New York, NY, and additional mailing offices. Subscription prices are $225 per year for (US individuals), $279 per year for (US institutions), $107 per year for (US students and residents), $253 per year for (Canadian individuals), $312 per year for (Canadian institutions), $269 per year for (international individuals), $312 per year for (international institutions), and $129 per year for (Canadian and foreign students/residents). To receive student/resident rate, orders must be accompanied by name of affiliated institution, date of term, and the signature of program/residency coordinator on institution letterhead. Orders will be billed at individual rate until proof of status is received. Foreign air speed delivery is included in all Clinics subscription prices. All prices are subject to change without notice. **POSTMASTER:** Send address changes to *Ultrasound Clinics,* Elsevier Health Sciences Division, Subscription Customer Service, 3251 Riverport Lane, Maryland Heights, MO 63043. **Customer Service (orders, claims, online, change of address): Telephone: 1-800-654-2452 (U.S. and Canada); 314-447-8871 (outside U.S. and Canada). Fax: 314-447-8029. E-mail: journalscustomerservice-usa@elsevier.com (for print support); journalsonlinesupport-usa@elsevier.com (for online support).**

Reprints: For copies of 100 or more, of articles in this publication, please contact the Commercial Reprints Department, Elsevier Inc., 360 Park Avenue South, New York, NY 10010-1710. Tel.: (+1) 212-633-3812; Fax: (+1) 212-462-1935; E-mail: reprints@elsevier.com.

Printed and bound by CPI Group (UK) Ltd, Croydon, CR0 4YY

Transferred to Digital Print 2011

Contributors

CONSULTING EDITOR

VIKRAM DOGRA, MD
Professor of Radiology, Urology, and
Biomedical Engineering, Director of Ultrasound
and Associate Chair for Education and
Research, Department of Imaging Sciences,
University of Rochester School of Medicine
and Dentistry, Rochester, New York

GUEST EDITORS

DEBORAH RUBENS, MD
Professor, URMC, Department of Imaging
Sciences, University of Rochester Medical
Center, Rochester, New York

EDWARD G. GRANT, MD
Professor and Chairman, USC, Department of
Radiology, USC University Hospital, Keck
School of Medicine, Los Angeles, California

AUTHORS

CARL A. ABTS, RDMS
Research Sonographer, Department
of Radiology, University of Alabama
at Birmingham, Birmingham, Alabama

JOHN J. CRONAN, MD
Professor of Diagnostic Imaging, Department
of Diagnostic Imaging, The Warren Alpert
Medical School of Brown University,
Rhode Island Hospital, Providence,
Rhode Island

M. ROBERT DE JONG, RDMS, RVT
Radiology Technical Manager, Division
of Ultrasound, Johns Hopkins Hospital,
Baltimore, Maryland

ULRIKE M. HAMPER, MD, MBA
Professor of Radiology, Urology and
Pathology; Chief, Ultrasound Section, Division
of Ultrasound, Russell H. Morgan Department
of Radiology and Radiological Science, The
Johns Hopkins University School of Medicine,
Baltimore, Maryland

BEVERLY E. HASHIMOTO, MD
Section Head of Ultrasound, Director,
Noninvasive Vascular Laboratory,
Department of Radiology, Virginia Mason
Medical Center, Seattle, Washington

IGOR LATICH, MD
Fellow, Interventional Radiology,
Department of Diagnostic Radiology, Yale
University School of Medicine, New Haven,
Connecticut

MARK E. LOCKHART, MD, MPH
Professor, Department of Radiology,
University of Alabama at Birmingham,
Birmingham, Alabama

MYRON A. POZNIAK, MD, FACR
Professor of Radiology, Chief of CT,
Department of Radiology, University
of Wisconsin School of Medicine and
Public Health, Madison, Wisconsin

STEPHANIE A. REID, MD
Postdoctoral Fellow, Russell H. Morgan
Department of Radiology and Radiological
Science, The Johns Hopkins University
School of Medicine, Baltimore, Maryland

MICHELLE L. ROBBIN, MD
Professor, Department of Radiology,
University of Alabama at Birmingham,
Birmingham, Alabama

LESLIE M. SCOUTT, MD
Medical Director, Professor of Diagnostic
Radiology and Surgery, Ultrasound Service,
Non-Invasive Vascular Laboratory,
Department of Diagnostic Radiology,
Yale University School of Medicine,
New Haven, Connecticut

HEIDI R. UMPHREY, MD
Assistant Professor, Department of Radiology,
University of Alabama at Birmingham,
Birmingham, Alabama

GAURAV VIJ, MD
Department of Diagnostic Radiology, Yale
University School of Medicine, New Haven,
Connecticut

STEVEN Y. WANG, MD
Department of Diagnostic Radiology,
Yale University School of Medicine,
New Haven, Connecticut

Contents

Many mistakes may be circumvented with skilled vascular technologists, high-quality equipment, understanding the ICA and ECA waveforms, and incorporating color Doppler in the vascular interpretation.

Vascular access procedures and associated complications are a major cause of morbidity and increasing health care cost in patients undergoing hemodialysis. Preoperative sonographic evaluation can alter surgical planning and increase the success of autogenous arteriovenous fistulas (AVFs). Ultrasonography may serve as a surrogate for AVF maturation. Studies disagree whether close access monitoring with early detection and intervention improves access longevity. Evaluation of the problem AVF and the synthetic arteriovenous graft, assessing for stenosis or other treatable causes of AVF nonmaturation and graft dysfunction, has been described. This review describes sonographic approaches for hemodialysis access planning and subsequent access assessment.

Renovascular hypertension is the most common surgically treatable cause of hypertension and, if untreated, the end result may be renal failure. Doppler ultrasound is an inexpensive, noninvasive screening method for diagnosing renovascular hypertension. It provides anatomic and functional information in a single study, aiding clinicians in preoperative and postoperative assessment for potential intervention, without the risks of radiation, nephrotoxicity, or nephrogenic systemic fibrosis. Doppler ultrasound's main limitation is technical failure to visualize the entire length of the main renal arteries. In the future, the use of intravenous ultrasound contrast agents and elastography could reduce the rate of technical failure.

Sonography is an important diagnostic tool in postoperative liver transplantation for the diagnosis of vascular complications, suspected or unsuspected. Early diagnosis of vascular complications can improve graft and patient survival by allowing earlier treatment. This article focuses on the evaluation of liver transplant vascular complications with duplex Doppler ultrasound. Because of the range of normal appearances in the immediate postoperative liver transplant, the ability to recognize normal postoperative findings from true complications is critical for interpretation. These normal early postoperative findings, as well as a brief explanation of basic liver transplant surgical techniques, are also reviewed.

This article discusses conditions that may be suitable for imaging with Doppler ultrasound techniques. These conditions include median arcuate ligament syndrome, ovarian torsion, arteriovenous fistula and pseudoaneurysm, air in the portal vein, aortic dissection, splenic artery aneurysm, coarctation of the aorta, asymmetric waveforms in the left and right hepatic arteries, hepatic arteriovenous malformations, and renal artery embolus.

Ultrasound Clinics

THE CLINICS ARE NOW AVAILABLE ONLINE!

Access your subscription at:
www.theclinics.com

GOAL STATEMENT
The goal of the *Ultrasound Clinics* is to keep practicing radiologists and radiology residents up to date with current clinical practice in ultrasound by providing timely articles reviewing the state of the art in patient care.

ACCREDITATION
The *Ultrasound Clinics* is planned and implemented in accordance with the Essential Areas and Policies of the Accreditation Council for Continuing Medical Education (ACCME) through the joint sponsorship of the University of Virginia School of Medicine and Elsevier. The University of Virginia School of Medicine is accredited by the ACCME to provide continuing medical education for physicians.

The University of Virginia School of Medicine designates this enduring material activity for a maximum of 15 *AMA PRA Category 1 Credit*(s)™ for each issue, 60 credits per year. Physicians should claim only the credit commensurate with the extent of their participation in the activity.

The American Medical Association has determined that physicians not licensed in the US who participate in this CME enduring material activity are eligible for a maximum of 15 *AMA PRA Category 1 Credit*(s)™ for each issue, 60 credits per year.

Credit can be earned by reading the text material, taking the CME examination online at http://www.theclinics.com/home/cme, and completing the evaluation. After taking the test, you will be required to review any and all incorrect answers. Following completion of the test and evaluation, your credit will be awarded and you may print your certificate.

FACULTY DISCLOSURE/CONFLICT OF INTEREST
The University of Virginia School of Medicine, as an ACCME accredited provider, endorses and strives to comply with the Accreditation Council for Continuing Medical Education (ACCME) Standards of Commercial Support, Commonwealth of Virginia statutes, University of Virginia policies and procedures, and associated federal and private regulations and guidelines on the need for disclosure and monitoring of proprietary and financial interests that may affect the scientific integrity and balance of content delivered in continuing medical education activities under our auspices.

The University of Virginia School of Medicine requires that all CME activities accredited through this institution be developed independently and be scientifically rigorous, balanced and objective in the presentation/discussion of its content, theories and practices.

All authors/editors participating in an accredited CME activity are expected to disclose to the readers relevant financial relationships with commercial entities occurring within the past 12 months (such as grants or research support, employee, consultant, stock holder, member of speakers bureau, etc.). The University of Virginia School of Medicine will employ appropriate mechanisms to resolve potential conflicts of interest to maintain the standards of fair and balanced education to the reader. Questions about specific strategies can be directed to the Office of Continuing Medical Education, University of Virginia School of Medicine, Charlottesville, Virginia.

The faculty and staff of the University of Virginia Office of Continuing Medical Education have no financial affiliations to disclose.

The authors/editors listed below have identified no professional or financial affiliations for themselves or their spouse/partner:
Carl A. Abts, RDMS; John J. Cronan, MD; M. Robert De Jong, RDMS, RVT; Barton Dudlick, (Acquisitions Editor); Ulrike M. Hamper, MD, MBA; Igor Latich, MD; Stephanie A. Reid, MD; Deborah Rubens, MD (Guest Editor); Heidi R. Umphrey, MD; Gaurav Vij, MD; and Steven Y. Wang, MD.

The authors/editors listed below have identified the following professional or financial affiliations for themselves or their spouse/partner:
Matthew J. Bassignani, MD (Test Author) is on the Advisory Board/Committee for Nuance and Fuji Medical Systems.
Vikram S. Dogra, MD (Consulting Editor) is the editor for the Journal of Clinical Imaging Science.
Edward Grant, MD (Guest Editor) is an industry funded researcher for Bracco and is on the Advisory Board/Committee for Nuance and Toshiba.
Beverly E. Hashimoto, MD is a consultant and on the Advisory Committee/Board for General Electric Medical Systems, is a consultant for Philips Medical Systems and Advanced Imaging Technologies, and is an industry funded research/investigator for U Systems.
Mark E. Lockhart, MD, MPH receives partial salary as the Deputy Editor for the Journal of Ultrasound in Medicine.
Myron A. Pozniak, MD owns stock in Cellectar.
Michelle L. Robbin, MD is an industry funded researcher for Bracco and Phillips Ultrasound.
Leslie M. Scoutt, MD is a consultant and receives honoraria for developing and presenting lectures for Philips Healthcare.

Disclosure of Discussion of Non-FDA Approved Uses for Pharmaceutical Products and/or Medical Devices
The University of Virginia School of Medicine, as an ACCME provider, requires that all faculty presenters identify and disclose any off-label uses for pharmaceutical and medical device products. The University of Virginia School of Medicine recommends that each physician fully review all the available data on new products or procedures prior to clinical use.

TO ENROLL
To enroll in the Ultrasound Clinics Continuing Medical Education program, call customer service at 1-800-654-2452 or visit us online at www.theclinics.com/home/cme. The CME program is available to subscribers for an additional fee of $196.00.

Preface
Vascular Ultrasound

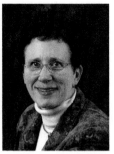 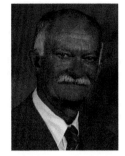

Deborah Rubens, MD   Edward G. Grant, MD
Guest Editors

The inaugural issue of *Ultrasound Clinics* in 2006 featured a section on Vascular Ultrasound as we felt it was one of the most valuable and unique diagnostic features of ultrasonic imaging. Subsequent issues on emergency imaging, abdominal imaging, and gynecological imaging have also included vascular articles to address specific organ-based disease processes. Five years later, ultrasound, and particularly vascular ultrasound, continues to grow in volume and complexity. Our initial monograph stressed the foundations of vascular ultrasound, Doppler artifacts and pitfalls, carotid and gynecologic imaging, as well as some more specialized articles on transcranial Doppler and Doppler imaging of arterial injuries. In this issue, we expand on that base with some more current and controversial topics. We review the technique as well as the pitfalls and controversies of lower and upper extremity deep venous thrombosis imaging, discuss the pitfalls of carotid imaging in general and specifically address carotid intimal hyperplasia, assess our role in dialysis vascular access, renal hypertension, and liver transplantation, and complete the issue with a case-based review of Doppler imaging in challenging abdominal cases.

Thanks to Dr Vikram Dogra, Consulting Editor, and to Barton Dudlick, our publisher, for their vision and faith in *Ultrasound Clinics*. Thanks to all of our contributors for their excellent articles. Thanks to the sonographers who create wonderful images and make outstanding ultrasound diagnoses daily.

We are sure that you, our readers, share our excitement and enthusiasm for this wonderful modality and the insight and information it brings us to care for our patients. We hope you find this issue valuable and helpful as well.

Deborah Rubens, MD
Department of Imaging Sciences
University of Rochester Medical Center
601 Elmwood Avenue, Box 648
Rochester, NY 14642, USA

Edward G. Grant, MD
Department of Radiology
USC University Hospital
Keck School of Medicine
1500 San Pablo Street
Los Angeles, CA 90033, USA

E-mail addresses:
Deborah_Rubens@URMC.Rochester.edu
(D. Rubens)
edgrant@usc.edu (E.G. Grant)

Ultrasound Clin 6 (2011) ix
doi:10.1016/j.cult.2011.09.001
1556-858X/11/$ – see front matter © 2011 Elsevier Inc. All rights reserved.

Deep Vein Thrombosis: Imaging Diagnosis and Related Controversies

John J. Cronan, MD

KEYWORDS

• DVT diagnosis • Venous ultrasound • Pulmonary embolus

Clot formation developing in the deep veins of the extremities (in most instances the focus is the lower extremity) is often a cause of local symptoms such as pain, swelling, and edema. In the long term, this clot formation can damage valves and ultimately lead to chronic venous insufficiency. However, in the acute setting, this fresh clot propagating in the venous system can break off and travel to the pulmonary arteries causing pulmonary embolus (PE). The frequency of PE is unknown. The size of the clot load traveling to the lung combined with the cardiopulmonary status of the patient determines the resulting symptomatic state. The spectrum of clinical manifestation extends from the asymptomatic state at one extreme to sudden death at the other.

In the past quarter century, venous ultrasonography has established itself as the dominant technique for evaluation of deep vein thrombosis (DVT). It is the gold standard. The prior diagnostic standard, venography, is rarely performed today and has inherent limitations, which led to its displacement.

The understanding of DVT and PE remains incomplete. The more these conditions are investigated, the more they lead to additional questions. In this sea of uncertainty, many issues regarding the diagnosis of DVT are unsettled, providing fertile environment for controversy. In this article, I review the present understanding and emphasize the controversies surrounding the imaging diagnosis of DVT. Much is to be learned, and knowing the controversial issues will accelerate this understanding.

RISK ASSESSMENT: WHO NEEDS TO BE STUDIED

The knowledge of the causation of DVT is expanding, revealing the ignorance regarding the cause of venous thrombosis. A recognizable cause for DVT is evident in nearly 70% of cases.[1] The knowledge gap is illustrated in the 30% of patients in whom no known risk factor is apparent.

Most imagers are familiar with the established causes of DVT: immobilization, trauma, pregnancy, and childbirth, as well as malignancy.[2,3] The relationship between estrogen and DVT has been established for more than 25 years.[4] In the past decade, mutations and conditions associated with thrombophilia have been defined, such as antithrombin, protein C or protein S, or factor V Leiden deficiency; prothrombin G20210A mutation; hyperhomocystinuria; and lupus anticoagulants.[5,6]

More recently, a link between DVT and atherosclerosis has been established.[1] The actual etiologic relationship is uncertain, but a diffuse underlying inflammation involving both the arterial and venous systems is suggested. There is confirmation of a relationship between asymptomatic atherosclerotic lesions and spontaneous venous thrombosis of the legs.

Eventually, all cases of DVT will have a definable etiology. At present, it is important that the

The author has nothing to disclose.
Department of Diagnostic Imaging, The Warren Alpert Medical School of Brown University, Rhode Island Hospital, 593 Eddy Street, Providence, RI 02903, USA
E-mail address: jcronan@lifespan.org

Ultrasound Clin 6 (2011) 421–433
doi:10.1016/j.cult.2011.07.002
1556-858X/11/$ – see front matter © 2011 Elsevier Inc. All rights reserved.

clinician be aware of the many causes and realize that unless they are identified and corrected, repeat episodes of DVT will occur. In fact, the repetitive nature of the thromboembolic process is emphasized by the fact that a major risk factor for recurrent DVT is a prior episode of DVT.

In the acute clinical situation, an assessment of the risk of DVT needs to be made. Wells and Anderson[7] have organized the risk into a scoring system with the suspicion of DVT ranked as likely or unlikely (**Table 1**). D-dimer assessment is often used in low- and moderate-probability cases. If the results of D-dimer tests are negative, there is no need to use imaging techniques. When the results of D-dimer tests are positive, venous ultrasonography is recommended to search for clot. Anticoagulation is not a benign treatment option; rather, it is associated with significant bleeding complications. A high degree of certainty regarding the presence of thromboembolic disease should be present before accepting the risks associated with anticoagulation.

Venous ultrasonography is performed whenever the D-dimer test result is positive and/or whenever there is a high clinical suspicion for DVT. However, in clinical practice, D-dimer test often is not used because the venous ultrasonography is so readily available and results can be available before D-dimer results. No doubt a high number of venous ultrasound examinations with negative results are seen. It could raise suspicion if the venous ultrasound examination is inappropriately being used.[8] Although an increasing number of venous ultrasound examinations with negative results are encountered, the benign nature of the study and the relative inexpensive cost propel its use forward. Concern for cost containment is abandoned when confronted with the reality of malpractice claims and the potential risk of missing DVT/PE.

TECHNIQUE

Venous ultrasonography of the lower extremities was established as a diagnostic technique based on the collapse of the vein lumen and coaptation of the vein walls. Pressure applied by the transducer, sufficient to dimple the overlying skin, should be enough pressure to collapse the lumen of the normal vein. Excessive compression is not required in the normal situation and, in fact, indicates the presence of pathology (**Fig. 1**).[9]

Standards set by accreditation organizations require evaluation of the lower extremity deep veins from the groin to the distal popliteal and the beginning of the tibial-peroneal trunk. The examination should be performed with the patient in the supine position with the leg externally rotated and slightly flexed. A 3- to 10-MHz linear transducer is used. The vein should be compressed throughout its course and coaptation of the wall noted. Compression is best done in the transverse projection, but sagittal orientation is

Table 1
The Wells score for DVT

Clinical Characteristics		Points
Active cancer (patient receiving treatment of cancer within the previous 6 months or currently receiving palliative treatment)		+1
Paralysis, paresis, or recent plaster immobilization of the lower extremities		+1
Recently bedridden for 3 d or more or major surgery within the previous 12 wk requiring general or regional anesthesia		+1
Localized tenderness along the distribution of the deep venous system		+1
Entire leg swollen		+1
Calf swelling at least 3 cm larger than that on the asymptomatic side (measured 10 cm below tibial tuberosity)		+1
Pitting edema confined to the symptomatic leg		+1
Collateral superficial veins (nonvaricose)		+1
Previously documented DVT		+1
Alternative diagnosis at least as likely as DVT		−2
Total Score	Clinical Probability	Prevalence of DVT
<2 points	DVT unlikely	5.5% (95% CI: 3.8–7.6%)
≥2 points	DVT likely	27.9% (95% CI: 23.9–31.8%)

Abbreviation: CI, confidence interval.

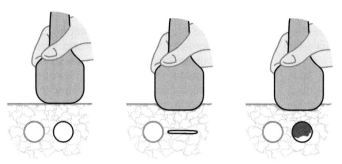

Fig. 1. Compression ultrasonography. (*Left*) Noncompression view of normal vein. Middle compression view of normal vein. (*Right*) compression view of acute occlusion of the vein. Note the lumen cannot be compressed because of the venous clot.

often used to document venous anatomy. Compression of the overlying skin should be sufficient to cause the normal vein to collapse. This amount of pressure would be approximately the same as pressing a bathroom scale to register 3 to 4 lb. In the normal setting, transducer pressure dimples the overlying skin. It is not possible to collapse the vein containing acute clot without excessive pressures, which will also collapse the accompanying artery (see **Fig. 1**).[9]

Color is used to demonstrate the presence of flow and use augmentation (compression of the leg muscles below the point of insonation) to demonstrate luminal patency indicated by increased flow when venous spectral Doppler waveforms interrogate the vein lumen. In addition, both femoral and iliac spectral waveforms should be evaluated for asymmetry or loss of respiratory phasicity.[10] The evaluation of the opposite leg waveform in the femoral/iliac region provides assessment of pelvis processes impeding venous blood flow.

When evaluating the upper extremity veins, the observation is compromised by the overlying clavicle, which prevents optimal interrogation of the vein and hinders the ability to compress the vein lumen (**Fig. 2**). Hence, compression is used when

possible, but investigators become reliant on the color flow and pulsed/spectral Doppler signal to interrogate the upper extremity veins.[10,11] Upper extremity evaluation consists of gray-scale and Doppler assessment of all accessible portions of the subclavian, innominate, internal jugular, and axillary veins. Compression is used whenever possible.[12] In addition, veins in the upper arm, that is, the basilic, cephalic, and brachial, should be evaluated to the elbow.

Any experienced sonographer can learn venous ultrasonography for assessment of DVT. I am somewhat concerned by the dispersion of ultrasonography throughout the medical community and use by those with no training. The extension of this concern has already occurred within the critical care community with the extrapolation that venous ultrasonography of the extremities can be performed by critical care physicians.[13]

TERMINOLOGY

Treatment of DVT is required when clot involves the deep veins. Involvement of the superficial, muscular, or perforating veins is not thought to generate sufficient risk of thromboembolic disease to justify the risks associated with anticoagulation. Saphenous clot within 2 cm of the femoral junction is deemed to be appropriate for anticoagulation.[14] Hence, it is very important to specify correctly and distinctly in reports the exact location of clot within the venous system.

Proper anatomic terminology in the venous system is important because many primary care physicians misconstrue venous ultrasonographic reports generated by radiologists. Radiologists have often identified the deep veins distal to the common femoral as the deep femoral vein and the superficial femoral vein. This identification can create confusion because the superficial femoral vein is actually a component of the deep venous system. A thrombus in this location requires treatment. When this venous segment is

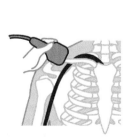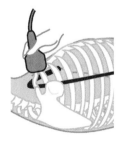

Fig. 2. Upper extremity venous evaluation. Anteroposterior (*left*) and lateral views (*right*) of upper extremity at the level of the clavicle. Note how the clavicle blocks complete visualization of the underlying vein.

labeled as superficial, a clinician unfamiliar with the terminology might assume that it is not an important vein (because it is a superficial vein) and decide not to initiate treatment.

To clarify this situation, the suggestion has been made that the femoral vein be called the femoral vein throughout its length (**Fig. 3**).[15] A permissible alternative is to refer to that portion of the femoral vein below the inguinal ligament and before the bifurcation as the common femoral vein. This confusing terminology is certainly worth avoiding because it would be unfortunate for a casual definition of venous anatomy to prevent a patient from being appropriately treated.

HOW MUCH OF THE LOWER EXTREMITY VEINS NEED TO BE STUDIED

Proper technique for ultrasound evaluation of the vein, as stated both in the American College of Radiology (ACR) standards in 1993 (revised in 2010) in collaboration with the American Institute of Ultrasound in Medicine and the Society of Radiologists in Ultrasound, indicates that a patient with a symptomatic extremity should be evaluated from the level of the inguinal ligament to the popliteal fossa in as continuous a manner as possible.[16] This includes all of the popliteal vein extending to the take off of the tibial-peroneal trunk.

It has been demonstrated that symptomatic patients have lengthy thrombi involving 1 or more venous segments.[17,18] Symptomatic thrombus usually involves multiple venous segments because it presents with a long clot. This presentation is different from the focal/isolated thrombi, which develop in the asymptomatic high-risk patients. In asymptomatic patients, thrombus often develops focally on valve cusps (**Fig. 4**).[19] This observation was demonstrated in a retrospective review of venograms and has been confirmed in the author's ultrasound laboratory. The author's group demonstrated that in approximately 99% of symptomatic cases, evaluation of the femoral or popliteal vein, using the 2-point compression technique, detects thrombus that extends above the knee. This 2-point evaluation requires only examination of the common femoral and popliteal venous areas (**Fig. 5**).[20]

This very abbreviated study detects a high percentage of cases with DVT. The overall decrease in the examination time is slightly in excess of 50%. Others who have demonstrated that approximately 95.4% of thrombus would be detected using a 2-point compression technique have confirmed the potential of the 2-point technique.[21] Obviously, there is some degree of compromise with the 2-point technique, balancing simplicity versus accuracy. This limited compression technique is not the accepted standard within the

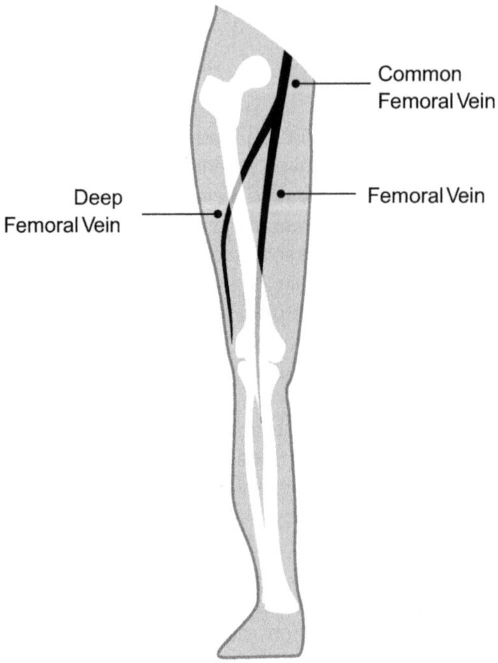

Fig. 3. Correct terminology of the femoral vein anatomy.

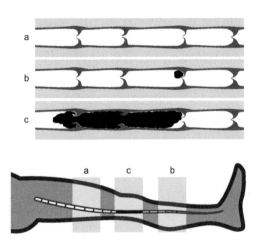

Fig. 4. Origin of venous clot in the lower extremities (a) Normal anatomy depicting the vein cusps (b) Asymptomatic focal clot on cusp. (c) Symptomatic state results when the focal clot promulgates. Leg schematic shows normal cusps and vein (a) in the thigh, asymptomatic focal small clot on valve cusp in the calf (b) and clot that has filled the lumen at the level of the popliteal vein (c).

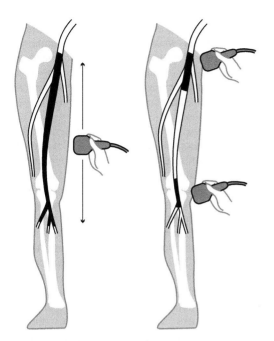

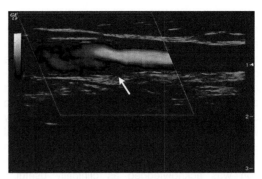

Fig. 6. Color Doppler depicting focal venous valve clot (*arrow*).

Fig. 5. Standard evaluation of lower extremity venous anatomy versus the 2-point evaluation. (*Left*) In the standard evaluation, the vein is studied in continuity from the inguinal ligament to the distal popliteal region, including the trifurcation (*darkened area*). (*Right*) Only the femoral and popliteal regions at a point are evaluated. This requires only 2 points of compression.

radiologic community in North America. However, the 2-point compression has utility in the emergency department or when evaluating the patient with extremely restricted mobility. In fact, the emergency medicine community has adopted the 2-point technique for the point of service examinations used by emergency room physicians.[22–24] Similarly, in Europe, the 2-point compression technique linked to the D-dimer laboratory test results is a standard approach for assessment. As an alternative to evaluating the entire leg, this 2-point technique provides an equivalent degree of certainty.[24,25] The literature supports a 2-point examination combined with D-dimer test as an equivalent study (see **Fig. 5**).[26]

THE CALF VEINS: A QUAGMIRE

Thrombi are most likely to develop in the small veins of the calf (see **Fig. 4**). In asymptomatic patients, thrombi form on valve cusps/pockets in a nearly routine manner. Valve pocket thrombi occur without any injury and are associated with stasis and immobility (**Fig. 6**).[27] I surmise that these tiny 1- to 2-mm clots break off from the valve

cusps as the patient assumes an upright position and begins ambulation.[28] These tiny clots within the pulmonary arteries have no clinical impact because they are too small to contribute to the clot load and induce a symptomatic state.[29,30] It is these tiny clots that embolize to the subsegmental branches of the pulmonary arteries and cause dotlike filling defects. With the improved resolution of multidetector computed tomography (MDCT), these incidental and asymptomatic clots are now seen in 3% to 5% of routine chest computed tomographies (CTs).[31–34] The ability to detect these small 1- to 2-mm clots on the valve cusps with routine ultrasonography is low. In fact, the venous ultrasonography usually has negative results if performed when a dot is the basis of the diagnosis of PE on the MDCT study.[35] When venous ultrasonography is held to the standard of being able to see these small clots in asymptomatic patients, it performs poorly. However, when patients have symptoms, investigators are looking for a more substantive clot load. In this setting, ultrasonography performs very well (see **Fig. 4**).

All ultrasonography accrediting organizations agree that when calf symptoms exist, direct evaluation of the calf, looking for the cause of calf discomfort, is necessary.[16,36] In this setting, investigators are looking for thrombus filling a lumen, causing inflammation and presenting as thromboembolic disease. As previously mentioned, calf clot can indeed embolize to the lung. In the setting of PE, clot is found in the calf veins only when calf symptoms exist.[37] Studies indicate that at least 20% to 30% of patients with calf clot produce nonclinical embolic disease. In the noncompromised patient, the clot load produced by these small vein thrombi/emboli is insufficient to cause pulmonary symptoms and clinical suspicion of PE.

The clinical acceptance of venous ultrasonography as a diagnostic technique in the evaluation of the symptomatic patient occurred based on clinical series that did not attempt direct evaluation of calf veins.[9,38] Indeed, the ultrasonographic units available in the early 1980s lacked probes with resolution to interrogate the small veins of the calf. In addition, color Doppler was not a component of these units, and initial validation was based on compression. The initial reports and literature describing the success of venous ultrasonography were based only on the evaluation of the femoral and popliteal veins. It was with this examination format that the compression ultrasound examination was acknowledged as clinically useful.[38] Although calf thrombi are common, they rarely cause acute clinical problems or clinical symptoms, and the validation of ultrasonography occurred without calf assessment.[39]

Eighty-eight percent of calf thrombus occurs in the asymptomatic patient (1- to 2-mm thrombus on a valve cusp), and this accounts for 50% of thrombi in the asymptomatic population. Similarly, the presence of calf thrombus is unlikely to lead to clinically significant PE.[40] PEs occur quietly and more frequently than we are aware. As pointed out by Moser and LeMoine,[41] patients with calf thrombus are unlikely to have signs or symptoms of PE. Pulmonary embolism that originates from the calf is usually asymptomatic because of the small clot load. Alternatively, patients with above-knee thrombus have PE in more than 50% of cases, despite the fact that they may not have any signs or symptoms of this phenomenon and evidence of PE is detected only on ventilation/perfusion scans, CT pulmonary arteriography, or pulmonary arteriograms.[42–44]

The knowledge of calf vein clot and its clinical impact remains in flux. However, a 2-front view of the process is being developed.[45,46] If thrombus is isolated to the calf veins, it seems to have little or no clinical impact in the acute setting. Calf clot does not cause clinically significant DVT/PE. The 3-month outcome when calf veins are evaluated and the calf clot is treated is equivalent to the clinical outcome when the calf veins are not interrogated.[26,47,48] The risk of anticoagulation is significant and, in many circles, is deemed to outweigh the value of treating acute calf clot.[25]

From the long-term chronic perspective, the issue now swings toward diagnosis and treatment of calf clot because data suggest a lower recurrence rate and decreased percentage of chronic venous insufficiency when the acute clot is initially treated at the time of diagnosis. The impetus of immediate treatment is from the recommendation of the American College of Chest Physicians.[49] Hence, the option of evaluating the calf at the time of the acute event may well be justified just to prevent chronic venous disease. If no clot is seen, no further study is necessary.[50–52] However, if a complete evaluation of the entire leg was not performed, as when a 2-point examination is done, one needs to reevaluate the proximal veins within a week or confirm a negative D-dimer result at the time of the initial study.[26,53,54] This algorithm prevents calf clot migration from moving into the proximal veins.[25]

Just as the clinical value of detecting calf clot is debatable, therapeutic management of patients with documented calf thrombus is similarly controversial.[44,55] Some suggest that observation of the acute calf thrombus with serial ultrasonographic studies is all that is necessary. A second examination, performed at 3 to 5 days from the baseline study, detects any upward propagation of calf vein thrombus into the popliteal system, and, if this occurs, treatment begins. However, the concern with the acceptance of this conservative approach is the evidence that patients with suspicion of calf thrombus do not return for a follow-up study.[56] Others strongly believe that therapy should be initiated at the initial presentation and argue that the potential for pulmonary embolism and the development of chronic venous insufficiency mandates anticoagulation.[41–44]

As mentioned previously, the issue that may well endorse the importance of evaluating the calf veins and treating calf thrombus relates to the development of chronic venous insufficiency.[57] Most venous valves are located below the knee. If thrombus develops in the calf area, irrespective of any risk to embolize, this clot leads to destruction of the calf vein valves and initiates chronic venous insufficiency. Therefore, logic strongly endorses direct evaluation of the calf veins to search for thrombus. Detection of thrombus permits treatment to be initiated so that the extent of valve destruction in the calf veins is minimized. Anticoagulation discourages the development of new clot; however, only a thrombolytic drug lyses the clot already developed.

This belief that calf thrombus embolizes and produces valve destruction is a forceful argument to support early diagnosis and treatment of thrombus isolated to calf veins.[58–61] The argument for direct calf evaluation, however, is countered with the risk of anticoagulation and the data showing that 3-month outcomes are the same with or without evaluation of the distal veins.[26,45]

Muscular veins of the calf, the gastrocnemius and soleal veins, are easily visualized in most patients.[46] These veins are not paired with an artery and, more importantly, are not deep veins. The deep veins run between muscles, and the muscular veins run within the muscles. Approximately 2% of symptomatic patients have muscular vein clot.

However, the implications of finding muscular vein clot in the calf are not clear. No treatment guidelines are available for this variant of DVT. There is no definitive proof that this clot should be treated in view of the risks of anticoagulation.[62–64] These muscle veins drain into the deep veins of the lower extremity. The soleal veins drain into the peroneal and posterior tibial veins, and the gastrocnemial veins drain into the popliteal veins. A recent series demonstrated 16% of clot in the muscular veins eventually extended into the tibial-peroneal system. Only 3% of isolated muscle vein clot extended into the popliteal vein, and this occurred within 15 days.[62]

Treatment standards for muscular clot are not established. Guidelines for assessment are not available. Based on limited data, a short course of anticoagulation is all that is necessary. One might withhold anticoagulation and reevaluate the muscular clot in 7 to 10 days to confirm the absence of migration.[48]

If a patient has signs or symptoms of calf thrombus, venous ultrasonography of the calf should be performed.[37] The presence of calf signs or symptoms necessitates a look at the calves because other disorders, such as calf hematoma, muscle rupture, or popliteal cyst, may be the cause of symptoms.

EVALUATION OF 1 OR 2 LEGS

In the era of venography, when the radiologist was requested to evaluate a patient for acute DVT, only the leg in question was studied.[65] Because of the risk of reactions to intravenous contrast material and the invasiveness of venography, the asymptomatic leg was not studied. Historically, noninvasive vascular laboratories using plethysmography routinely evaluated both the symptomatic and the asymptomatic leg. These laboratories, which are usually directed by surgeons, not radiologists, used the information obtained from the asymptomatic leg as a frame of reference to help diagnose any thrombus that might be present in the symptomatic leg. After the introduction of venous ultrasonography, radiologists continued to evaluate only the symptomatic leg. Alternatively, many vascular laboratories, which had developed a pattern of noninvasively evaluating both the symptomatic and the asymptomatic leg, continued this practice as the transition occurred from plethysmography to venous ultrasonography.

When a patient presents with unilateral symptoms, it is only necessary to evaluate the side with symptoms. There is a *Current Procedural Terminology* code for a unilateral examination. Controversy exists regarding the importance and

frequency of finding thrombus in the asymptomatic leg.[7,66,67] Historically, the literature has indicated that the asymptomatic leg does not harbor thrombus. More recently, articles have been published suggesting that thrombus can be found in the asymptomatic leg, but the frequency of this finding in a patient with a negative evaluation of the symptomatic leg occurred in less than 1% of cases.[68–70] Certainly, finding thrombus in the asymptomatic leg of a patient with thrombus in the symptomatic leg will not alter treatment. The likelihood of finding thrombus solely in the asymptomatic leg is between 0% and 1%. I suggest that this low frequency of thrombus does not justify a routine evaluation of the asymptomatic leg in a patient presenting with a single symptomatic extremity.[8]

Adding to the confusion regarding the unilateral examination has been the addition to the ACR guidelines in 2010.[16] It is now recommended that the femoral or iliac veins on both sides be interrogated with spectral Doppler waveforms to evaluate and confirm that phasicity is normal and symmetric. This recommendation is an effort to be more cognizant of uphill masses or partial obstruction in the pelvic veins. Although inherently a good recommendation, it created confusion regarding the need to evaluate the asymptomatic leg.

THE BILATERAL VENOUS EXAMINATION

With the lack of good objective clinical parameters to diagnose DVT, recommending a bilateral venous ultrasonography is increasing in frequency. However, this examination has the highest likelihood of being normal in my experience. The benign nature of the lower extremity venous examination encourages excess use. Unlike the days of venography when only a unilateral examination was performed because of discomfort, complexity, and risks, the lower extremity ultrasonography presents no such barriers. Most of these patients have cardiac or peripheral vascular disease as the cause of their symptoms.[70] It is extraordinarily rare for the results of these examinations to be positive, and this is most likely in the subgroup of oncology patients who have metastatic disease. Again, this is a situation in which assessment of the risks factors helps (see **Table 1**). However, I am a realist and understand that it is easier to recommend a bilateral examination than to consider the risk factors.[69–71]

SIGNIFICANCE OF A NEGATIVE EXAMINATION RESULT

Evidence exists that a compression ultrasonographic study of a symptomatic lower extremity with negative results, using complete evaluation of both the femoral and popliteal veins, provides sufficient validation to withhold anticoagulation.[68–72] The need for any follow-up studies in these cases is somewhat less well defined, but the evidence suggests that if the patient remains symptomatic, a repeat study of the lower extremity should be performed 3 to 5 days after the initial examination. An alternative proved technique to finalize the workup is to demonstrate a normal study of the proximal veins combined with a negative D-dimer result. Such a negative combination obviates the need to reassess the leg.[73] Theoretically, if silent calf clot exits,[73] small focal calf thrombi might propagate upward into the popliteal vein and cause symptoms. However, it is likely that the patient with isolated calf clot would have calf symptoms, which stimulate the direct evaluation of the calf and the focal area of pain. As has been mentioned previously, the potential for direct evaluation of the calf veins needs to be considered as a more direct approach to immediate diagnosis, and all accreditation groups suggest direct calf assessment of the calf when calf signs or symptoms exist.

ULTRASONOGRAPHY FOR THE ASSESSMENT OF PULMONARY EMBOLISM

With the acceptance of CT pulmonary angiography (CTPE) as the primary tool to look for pulmonary embolism, a great deal more patients are evaluated for PE. The incidence of pulmonary embolism has risen dramatically but without any change in the death rate.[31,74] This suggests that clots that have a low clinical impact and were not diagnosed previously are diagnosed. Adding to the confusion surrounding this issue is the concern for radiation and its long-term impact in the population.[75–77]

These factors have contributed to the continued and increasing use of bilateral lower extremity venous ultrasonography to look for DVT as a surrogate for PE. If DVT is diagnosed in either leg, treatment with anticoagulation is initiated and also treatment of PE is provided. The logic of this seems straightforward.[72] PE is caused by DVT. However, investigators have come to realize that not all PEs have demonstrable DVT. The initial questioning of this logic began 20 years ago when it was noted that only 70% of PE cases had venographically demonstrated DVT. With the diagnosis of greater numbers of small incidental clots and smaller clot loads in the pulmonary arteries, the percentage of patients with positive DVT continues to decrease. Recent data suggest that only 20% to 30% of patients with PE have

demonstrable DVT.[78] Lower extremity venous ultrasonography to assess for pulmonary embolism is most productive when leg signs or symptoms exist.[79–81] Importantly, clinicians need to understand that the absence of lower extremity DVT cannot be associated with the absence of PE. A ventilation-perfusion scan or MDCT needs to be performed to answer the clinical question regarding the presence or absence of PE.

Hence, the absence of lower extremity DVT cannot be used to exclude PE. In fact many have wondered if this surrogate diagnosis remains justified as a cost-effective technique in excluding PE.[82] Often, clinicians recommend lower extremity venous ultrasonography when PE has been visualized to assess the possible clot load remaining in the lower extremities. A large remaining clot load in the legs will be used to factor consideration for an inferior vena cava filter.

The venous ultrasound examination of the lower extremity in a setting of possible PE should be focused. In the absence of any symptoms or signs in the lower extremities, only the femoral-popliteal system needs to be evaluated. As discussed in the calf section, symptomatic PE from asymptomatic calf thrombus is very rare. A recent proposal has been to use CTPE in the workup of PE and to complement CT with compression ultrasonography.[83,84] The suggestion has been made that if a patient presents with symptoms of both DVT and PE, ultrasonography of the lower extremities should be obtained first. If the test result is positive for thrombus, treatment of venous thromboembolic disease should be initiated. A negative venous ultrasonography study result should be followed by CTPE to exclude PE via direct visualization of the pulmonary arteries. Either an MDCT scan demonstrating pulmonary artery thrombus or a compression ultrasonography demonstrating lower extremity DVT permits treatment to be started. Negative study results permit anticoagulation to be withheld.[85]

With this information, the question remains: where is PE coming from? Did the clot embolize in toto leaving nothing behind in the legs? What is the role of upper extremity clot? The literature suggests that up to 10% to 30% of PE originate in the upper extremities, but this is primarily in patients who have indwelling lines and catheters.[86,87] There have even been some recent suggestions that clot may form de novo in the pulmonary arteries.[88] This last theory seems a little excessive but exemplifies the struggle to explain the origin of PE.

With this background information, the question remains: where does PE come from. Lessons from medical school are not consistent with clinical practice. Malpractice cases are filed everyday based on a negative result of lower extremity ultrasonography and a patient dead 2 to 3 days later from a massive PE. Daily scan can be recommended in patients who have massive PE and in whom no clot can be found in the extremities. I am convinced that the more I learn about thromboembolic disease, the more questions are raised.

THE DIAGNOSIS OF DVT AND THE NEED FOR A FOLLOW-UP STUDY

After diagnosing DVT, the role of the follow-up examination frequently is raised. The need and role of a follow-up study depend on the question asked. It is a common occurrence that patients with a clear-cut DVT are sent back to the ultrasonography laboratory within 1 to 2 days of the initial diagnosis of DVT, with a request for a follow-up examination. The history accompanying the requisition notes concern for evaluation of clot propagation. However, clinicians often fail to realize that anticoagulation does not produce lysis of the clot already present in the extremity. In fact, studies have shown that approximately 40% of the clot actually propagates in the first few days after anticoagulation is started.[89] Adequately anticoagulated patients achieve clot stability at approximately 9 days. At this time, all free-floating clot should become attached to the vein wall and have no embolic potential.[90] Hence, there is no need to take a look at the acute clot and to evaluate for change. In my experience, the normal

propagation, which is reported, may only contribute to unneeded concern by the clinicians.

As the time of completion of anticoagulation approaches, a follow-up study does become a very reasonable idea.[91] Clot evolution is a dynamic process occurring over approximately 6 months (**Fig. 7**). At the 6-month mark approximately half of the affected veins return to a normal state with no evidence of prior clot.[92] These veins have a normal lumen, show blood flow filling the vein lumen, and have normal compression. Certain factors make this desirable outcome more likely: young age of the patient, short segment clot, and clot in a large vessel, which is not occlusive. Of the 50% of veins with residual abnormalities, the outcome can be (1) persistent total venous occlusion with complete filling of lumen with soft tissue or (2) recanalization of a smaller lumen with scar along the wall. In the second scenario, the new lumen compresses but the adherent scar reduces lumen size from that of the original. In both theses scenarios, the vein is not enlarged. In the acute scenario the size of the vein can swell and be more than twice the size of the accompanying artery. Even in the presence of focal scarring, the residual vein lumen is now compressible. The thrombophlebitis (inflammation of the vessel wall) has resolved over these 6 months, and the overall size of the vein is normal.

Ultrasound assessment at this 6-month postacute episode provides a new baseline regarding the status of the vein lumen. Physicians will know in which half of outcomes their patient resides, that is, if the vein is back to normal or does it

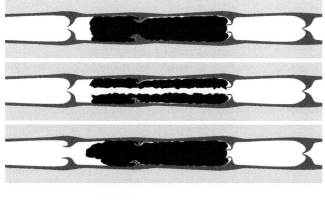
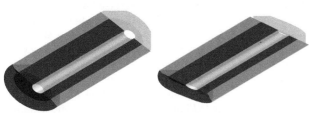

Fig. 7. Evolution of clot. If clot is followed from diagnosis to 6 months, half the patients return to normal. The others are left with residual scar. (*Top*) Total occlusion at time of initial diagnosis. (*Middle*) Partial recanalization with a decreased lumen at 6 months. (*Bottom*) Persistence of luminal occlusion by scar. The 2 cross-sectional images show that the recanalized lumen is seen to compress (*lower right*), but the scar limits the size of the lumen.

have residual disease.[92–94] It is important to avoid diagnosing these chronic changes because acute DVT, a misdiagnosis, is all too frequent.

The presence of residual disease or scarring in the lumen indicates those veins likely to experience venous insufficiency because of valve dysfunction (see **Fig. 7**). In addition, the observation of residual changes in the vein at 6 months indicates an increased risk of recurrent DVT. It is recommended that patients exhibiting these findings at the end of the anticoagulation period should have anticoagulation treatment continued.[95,96]

However, thrombosed veins that appear to completely recanalize may still develop valve incompetence and lead therefore to chronic venous insufficiency.[97]

SUMMARY

Venous ultrasonography has assumed an important role in the diagnosis of DVT/PE. Compression remains the dominant technique and can be easily performed by the experienced practitioner. Many controversies exist, but these are predominantly related to the lack of knowledge regarding DVT and the linkage of DVT with PE. It is important to understand these limitations so that proper patient care is provided.

REFERENCES

1. Prandoni P, Bilora F, Marchiori A, et al. An association between atherosclerosis and venous thrombosis. N Engl J Med 2003;348:1435–41.
2. Geerts WH, Code KI, Jay RM, et al. A prospective study of venous thromboembolism after major trauma. N Engl J Med 1994;331:1601–6.
3. Toglia MR, Weg JG. Venous thromboembolism during pregnancy. N Engl J Med 1996;335:108–14.
4. Vandenbroucke JP, Rosing J, Bloemenkamp KW, et al. Oral contraceptives and the risk of venous thrombosis. N Engl J Med 2001;344:1527–35.
5. Seligsohn U, Lubetsky A. Genetic susceptibility to venous thrombosis. N Engl J Med 2001;344:1222–31.
6. Den Heijer M, Koster T, Blom HJ, et al. Hyperhomocysteinemia as a risk factor for deep-vein thrombosis. N Engl J Med 1996;344:1527–35.
7. Wells PS, Anderson DR. Value of assessment of pretest probability of deep-vein thrombosis in clinical management. Lancet 1997;350:1795–8.
8. Fowl RJ, Strothman GB, Blebea J, et al. Inappropriate use of venous duplex scans: an analysis of indications and results. J Vasc Surg 1996;23:881–6.
9. Cronan JJ, Dorfman GS, Scola FH, et al. Deep venous thrombosis: US assessment using vein compression. Radiology 1987;162:191–4.
10. Selis JE, Kadakia S. Venous Doppler sonography of the extremities: a window to pathology of the thorax, abdomen and pelvis. AJR Am J Roentgenol 2009; 193:1446–51.
11. Patel MC, Berman LH, Moss HA, et al. Subclavian and internal jugular veins at Doppler US: abnormal cardiac pulsatility and respiratory phasicity as a predictor of complete central occlusion. Radiology 1999;211:579–83.
12. Chin EE, Zimmerman PT, Grant EG. Sonographic evaluation of upper extremity deep venous thrombosis. J Ultrasound Med 2005;24:829–38.
13. Kory PD, Pellecchia CM, Shiloh AL, et al. Accuracy of ultrasonography performed by critical care physicians for the diagnosis of deep venous thrombosis. Chest 2011;139(3):538–42. Available at: http://chestjournal. chestpubs.org.revproxy.brown.edu/content/early/2010/ 10/26/chest.10-1479.full.pdf+html?sid=b57e8f33-691f-40bb-a859-0961d1288a61. Accessed December 29, 2010.
14. Sover ER, Brammer HM, Rowedder AM. Thrombosis of the proximal greater saphenous vein: ultrasonographic diagnosis and clinical significance. J Ultrasound Med 1997;16:113–6.
15. Bundens WP, Bergan JJ, Halasz NA, et al. The superficial femoral vein: a potentially lethal misnomer. JAMA 1995;274:1296–8.
16. ACR-AIUM-SRU practice guideline for the performance of peripheral venous ultrasound examination. American College of Radiology website. Available at: http://www.acr.org/SecondaryMainMenuCategories/ quality_safety/guidelines/us/us_peripheral_venous. aspx. Accessed December 29, 2010.
17. Cogo A, Lensing AW, Prandoni P, et al. Distribution of thrombosis in patients with symptomatic deep vein thrombosis. Arch Intern Med 1993;153: 2777–80.
18. Markel A, Manzo RA, Bergelin RO, et al. Patterns and distribution of thrombi in acute venous thrombosis. Arch Surg 1992;127:305–9.
19. Rose SC, Swiebel WJ, Miller FJ. Distribution of acute lower extremity deep venous thrombosis in symptomatic and asymptomatic patients: imaging implications. J Ultrasound Med 1994;13:243–50.
20. Pezzullo JA, Perkins AB, Cronan JJ. Symptomatic deep vein thrombosis: diagnosis with limited compression US. Radiology 1996;198:67–70.
21. Frederick MG, Hertzberg BS, Kliewer MA, et al. Can the US examination for lower extremity deep venous thrombosis be abbreviated? A prospective study of 755 examinations. Radiology 1996;199:45–7.
22. Mattu A. Learn how to diagnose lower extremity deep venous thrombosis with beside emergency department ultrasound. In: Mattu A, Chanmugam AS, Swadron SP, et al, editors. Avoiding common errors in the emergency department. Philadelphia: Lippincott Williams & Wilkins; 2010. p. 696–9.

23. Ashar T, Jayarama K, Yun R. Bedside ultrasound for detection of deep vein thrombosis: the two-point compression method. ISRJEM 2006;6:36–43.

24. Jacoby J, Cesta M, Axelband J. Can emergency medicine residents detect acute deep venous thrombosis with a limited, two-site ultrasound examination? J Emerg Med 2007;32:197–200.

25. Landefeld CS. Noninvasive diagnosis of deep vein thrombosis. JAMA 2008;300:1696–7.

26. Bernardi E, Camporese G, Büller HR, et al. Serial 2-point ultrasonography plus D-dimer vs. whole-leg color-coded Doppler ultrasonography for diagnosing suspected symptomatic deep vein thrombosis. JAMA 2008;300:1653–9.

27. Sevitt S. The structure and growth of valve-pocket thrombi in femoral veins. J Clin Pathol 1974;27:517–28.

28. Suh JM, Cronan JJ, Healey TT. Dots are not clots: the over-diagnosis and over-treatment of PE. Emerg Radiol 2010;17:347–52.

29. Eyer BA, Goodman LR, Washington L. Clinicians' response to radiologists' reports of isolated subsegmental pulmonary embolism or inconclusive interpretation of pulmonary embolism using MDCT. AJR Am J Roentgenol 2005;184:623–8.

30. Stein PD, Hull RD, Raskob GE. Withholding treatment in patients with acute pulmonary embolism who have a high risk of bleeding and negative serial noninvasive leg tests. Am J Med 2000;109:301–6.

31. Burge AJ, Freeman KD, Klapper PJ, et al. Increased diagnosis of pulmonary embolism without a corresponding decline in mortality during the CT era. Clin Radiol 2008;63:381–6.

32. DeMonaco NA, Dang Q, Kapoor WN, et al. Pulmonary embolism incidence is increasing with use of spiral computed tomography. Am J Med 2008;121:611–7.

33. Anderson DR, Kahn SR, Rodger MA, et al. Computed tomographic pulmonary angiography vs. ventilation-perfusion lung scanning in patients with suspected pulmonary embolism. A randomized controlled trial. JAMA 2007;298:2743–53.

34. Goodman LR. Small pulmonary emboli: what do we know? Radiology 2005;234:654–8.

35. Le Gal G, Righini M, Parent F, et al. Diagnosis and management of subsegmental pulmonary embolism. J Thromb Haemost 2006;4:724–31.

36. Dorfman GS, Cronan JJ, Tupper TB, et al. Occult pulmonary embolism: a common occurrence in deep venous thrombosis. AJR Am J Roentgenol 1987;148:263–6.

37. Gottlieb RH, Voci SL, Syed L, et al. Randomized prospective study comparing routine versus selective use of sonography of the complete calf in patients with suspected deep venous thrombosis. AJR Am J Roentgenol 2003;180:241–5.

38. Vaccaro JP, Cronan JJ, Dorfman GS. Outcome analysis of patients with normal compression US examinations. Radiology 1990;175:645–9.

39. Gottlieb RH, Widjaja J, Mehra S, et al. Clinically important pulmonary emboli: does calf vein US alter outcomes? Radiology 1999;211:25–9.

40. Huisman MV, Büller HR, Ten Cate JW, et al. Serial impedance plethysmography for suspected deep venous thrombosis in outpatients. N Engl J Med 1986;314:823–8.

41. Moser KM, LeMoine JR. Is embolic risk conditioned by location of deep venous thrombosis? Ann Intern Med 1981;94:439–44.

42. Huisman MV, Büller HR, Ten Cate JW, et al. Unexpected high prevalence of silent pulmonary embolism in patients with deep venous thrombosis. Chest 1989;95:498–502.

43. Philbrick JT, Becker DM. Calf deep vein thrombosis: a wolf in sheep's clothing? Arch Intern Med 1988; 148:2131–8.

44. Lohr JM, Kerr TM, Lutter KS, et al. Lower extremity calf thrombosis: to treat or not to treat? J Vasc Surg 1991;14:618–23.

45. Righini M. Is it worth diagnosing and treating distal deep vein thrombosis? No. J Thromb Haemost 2007;5:55–9.

46. Schellong SM. Distal DVT: worth diagnosing? Yes. J Thromb Haemost 2007;5:51–4.

47. Büller HR, Arina J, ten Cate-Hook AJ, et al. Safely ruling out deep venous thrombosis in primary care. Ann Intern Med 2009;150:229–35.

48. Righini M, Bounameux H. Clinical relevance of distal deep vein thrombosis. Curr Opin Pulm Med 2008; 14:408–13.

49. Kearon C, Kahn SR, Agnelli G, et al. Antithrombotic therapy for venous thromboembolic disease: American College of Chest Physicians evidence-based clinical practical guidelines (8th edition). Chest 2008;133: 454S–545S.

50. Schellong SM. Venous ultrasonography in symptomatic and asymptomatic patients: an updated review. Curr Opin Pulm Med 2008;14:374–80.

51. Friera A, Giménez NR, Caballero P, et al. Deep vein thrombosis? Can a second sonographic examination be avoided? AJR Am J Roentgenol 2002;178: 1001–5.

52. Subramaniam RM, Heath R, Chou T, et al. Deep venous thrombosis: withholding anticoagulation therapy after negative complete lower limb US findings. Radiology 2005;237:348–52.

53. Bernardi E, Prandoni P, Lensing AW, et al. D-dimer testing as an adjunct to ultrasonography in patients with clinically suspected deep vein thrombosis: prospective cohort study. BMJ 1998;317:1037–40.

54. Johnson SA, Stevens SM, Woller SC. Risk of deep vein thrombosis following a single negative whole-leg compression ultrasound. JAMA 2010;303:438–45.

55. Solis MM, Ranval TJ, Nix ML, et al. Is anticoagulation indicated for asymptomatic postoperative calf vein thrombosis? J Vasc Surg 1992;16:414–9.

56. McIlrath ST, Blaivas M, Lyon M. Patient follow-up after negative lower extremity bedside ultrasound for deep venous thrombosis in the ED. Am J Emerg Med 2006;24:325–8.

57. Masuda EM, Kessler DM, Kistner RL, et al. The natural history of calf vein thrombosis: lysis of thrombi and development of reflux. J Vasc Surg 1998;28:67–74.

58. Kakkar VV, Howe CT, Flane C, et al. Natural history of postoperative deep venous thrombosis. Lancet 1969;2:230–2.

59. Langerstedt CL, Olsson CG, Fagher BO, et al. Need for long-term anticoagulant treatment in symptomatic calf vein thrombosis. Lancet 1985;2:515–8.

60. Cornuz J, Pearson SD, Polak JF. Deep venous thrombosis: complete lower extremity venous US examination in patients without known risk factors—outcome study. Radiology 1999;211:637–41.

61. Atri M, Herva MJ, Reinhold C, et al. Accuracy of sonography in the evaluation of calf deep vein thrombosis in both postoperative surveillance and symptomatic patients. AJR Am J Roentgenol 1996; 166:1361–7.

62. MacDonald PS, Kahn SR, Miller N, et al. Short-term natural history of isolated gastrocnemius and soleal vein thrombosis. J Vasc Surg 2003;37:523–7.

63. Schwartz T, Schmidt B, Beyer J, et al. Therapy of isolated calf muscle vein thrombosis with low-molecular-weight heparin. Blood Coagul Fibrinolysis 2001;12:597–9.

64. Lautz TB, Abbas F, Novis Walsh SJ, et al. Isolated gastrocnemius and soleal vein thrombosis: should these patients receive therapeutic anticoagulation? Ann Surg 2010;251:735–42.

65. Cronan JJ. Deep venous thrombosis: one leg or both legs? Radiology 1996;200:323–4.

66. Sheiman RG, McArdle CR. Bilateral lower extremity US in the patient with unilateral symptoms of deep venous thrombosis: assessment of need. Radiology 1995;194:171–3.

67. Strotham G, Blebea J, Fowl RJ, et al. Contralateral duplex scanning for deep venous thrombosis is unnecessary in patients with symptoms. J Vasc Surg 1995;22:543–7.

68. Cronan JJ. Controversies in venous ultrasound. Semin Ultrasound CT MR 1997;18:33–8.

69. Naidich JB, Torre JR, Pellerito JS, et al. Suspected deep venous thrombosis: is US of both legs necessary? Radiology 1996;200:429–31.

70. Sheiman RG, Weintrub JL, McArdle CR. Bilateral lower extremity US in the patient with bilateral symptoms of deep venous thrombosis: assessment of need. Radiology 1995;196:379–81.

71. Anderson FA, Wheeler HB. Physician priorities in the management of venous thromboembolism: a community wide survey. J Vasc Surg 1992;15:707–14.

72. Cronan JJ. Venous thromboembolic disease: the role of US. Radiology 1993;186:619–30.

73. Kearon C, Ginsberg JS, Douketis J, et al. A randomized trial of diagnostic strategies after normal proximal vein ultrasonography for suspected deep venous thrombosis: D-dimer testing compared with repeated ultrasonography. Ann Intern Med 2005;142:490–6.

74. Auer RC, Schulman AR, Tuorto S, et al. Use of helical CT is associated with an increased incidence of postoperative pulmonary emboli in cancer patients with no change in the number of fatal pulmonary emboli. J Am Coll Surg 2009;208:871–80.

75. Brenner DJ, Hall EJ. Computed tomography—an increasing source of radiation exposure. N Engl J Med 2007;357:2277–84.

76. Einstein AJ, Henzlova MJ, Rajagopalan S. Estimating risk of cancer associated with radiation exposure from 64-slice computed tomography coronary angiography. JAMA 2007;298:317–23.

77. Killewich LA, Nunnelee JD, Auer AI. Value of lower extremity venous duplex examination in the diagnosis of pulmonary embolism. J Vasc Surg 1993;17:934–9.

78. Konstantinides S. Acute pulmonary embolism. N Engl J Med 2008;359:2804–13.

79. Turkstra F, Kuijer PM, van Beek EJR, et al. Diagnostic utility of ultrasonography of leg veins in patients suspected of having pulmonary embolism. Ann Intern Med 1997;126:775–81.

80. Sheiman RG, McArdle CR. Clinically suspected pulmonary embolism: use of bilateral lower extremity US as the initial examination—a prospective study. Radiology 1999;212:75–8.

81. MacGilavry MR, Sanson B, Büller HR, et al. Compression ultrasonography of the leg veins in patients with clinically suspected pulmonary embolism. Is a more extensive assessment of compressibility useful? Thromb Haemost 2000;84:973–6.

82. Righini M, Le Gal G, Aujesky D, et al. Diagnosis of pulmonary embolism by multidetector CT alone or combined with venous ultrasonography of the leg: a randomized non-inferiority trial. Lancet 2008;371: 1343–52.

83. Rosen MP, Sheiman RG, Weintraub J, et al. Compression sonography in patients with indeterminate or low-probability lung scans: lack of usefulness in the absence of both symptoms of deep vein thrombosis and thromboembolic risk factors. AJR Am J Roentgenol 1996;166:285–9.

84. Hull RD, Hirsh J, Carter CJ, et al. Pulmonary angiography, ventilation lung scanning, and venography for clinically suspected pulmonary embolism with abnormal perfusion lung scan. Ann Intern Med 1983;98:891–9.

85. Goodman LR, Lipchik RJ. Diagnosis of acute pulmonary embolism: time for a new approach. Radiology 1996;199:25–7.

86. Mustafa S, Stein PD, Patel KC, et al. Upper extremity deep venous thrombosis. Chest 2003;123:1953–6.

87. Prandoni P, Polistena P, Bernardi E, et al. Upper-extremity deep vein thrombosis. Risk factors, diagnosis and complications. Arch Intern Med 1997; 157:57–62.

88. Schultz DJ, Brasel KJ, Washington L, et al. Incidence of asymptomatic pulmonary embolism in moderately to severely injured trauma patients. J Trauma 2004;56:727–33.

89. Krupski WC, Bass A, Dilley RB, et al. Propagation of deep venous thrombosis identified by duplex ultrasonography. J Vasc Surg 1990;12:467–75.

90. Berry RE, George JE, Shaver WA. Free-floating deep venous thrombosis. Ann Surg 1990;211:719–23.

91. Cronan JJ, Leen V. Recurrent deep venous thrombosis: limitations of US. Radiology 1989;170:739–42.

92. Murphy TP, Cronan JJ. Evolution of deep venous thrombosis: a prospective evaluation with US. Radiology 1990;177:543–8.

93. Prandoni JA, Arcelus JU, Hoffman KN, et al. A simple ultrasound approach for detection of recurrent proximal-vein thrombosis. Circulation 1993;88:1730–5.

94. Caprini JA, Arcelus JI, Hoffman KN, et al. Venous duplex imaging follow-up of acute symptomatic deep vein thrombosis of the leg. J Vasc Surg 1995;21:472–6.

95. Prandoni P, Prins MH, Lensing AW, et al. Residual thrombosis on ultrasonography to guide the duration of anticoagulation in patients with deep venous thrombosis. Ann Intern Med 2009;150:577–85.

96. Siragusa S, Malato A, Anastasio R, et al. Residual vein thrombosis to establish duration of anticoagulation after a first episode of deep vein thrombosis: the Duration of Anticoagulation based on Compression Ultra-Sonography (DACUS) study. Blood 2008;112:511–5.

97. Killewich LA, Bedford GR, Beach KW, et al. Spontaneous lysis of deep venous thrombi: rate and outcome. J Vasc Surg 1989;9:89–97.

Upper Extremity Venous Doppler

Myron A. Pozniak, MD

KEYWORDS

- Upper extremity • Deep vein thrombosis
- Ultrasound • Doppler

Ultrasonography is a noninvasive and reliable method for examining the upper extremity (UE) venous system, particularly with respect to the diagnosis or exclusion of thrombus in symptomatic patients.[1] Indeed, the most frequent indication for ultrasonography of the UE veins is to evaluate for deep vein thrombosis (DVT).

Upper extremity deep vein thrombosis (UEDVT) generally arises in the presence of recognizable risk factors, such as with central venous catheters inserted for intensive care monitoring, chemotherapy, dialysis, or parenteral feeding. Cancer patients who develop a hypercoagulable state are also at greater risk. As many as 20% of patients, however, present spontaneously with no recognizable risk factors (**Box 1**).

To accurately exclude the presence of DVT the UE ultrasound examination requires knowledge of standard venous anatomy, proper b-mode imaging and Doppler technique, and recognition of normal and abnormal Doppler waveforms.

UPPER EXTREMITY VENOUS ANATOMY

As in the leg, the venous system of the UE is divided into deep and superficial vessels. The distal deep veins are paired and accompany the arteries: radial and ulnar. More proximally the venous system continues as the brachial, axillary, subclavian, and brachiocephalic veins. The cephalad extent of vein pairing is variable. Most patients have single brachial veins, but pairing can be seen to extend to involve the axillary veins (**Fig. 1**). Communication among the veins of the deep system is variable.

The UE superficial venous system is more variable than in the leg, but there are two main channels: the cephalic vein along the radial aspect of the arm and the basilic vein along the ulnar side (**Fig. 2**). These veins communicate at the antecubital fossa via the median antecubital vein. The basilic vein pierces the deep fascia on the medial aspect of the mid-upper arm to merge with the brachial vein, and this combined channel becomes the axillary vein as it enters the axilla. The cephalic vein passes more cephalad along the lateral aspect of the biceps. At the level of pectoralis major it courses medially and deeply to pierce the clavipectoral fascia below the clavicle, and joins the axillary vein. Other tributaries from the region of the shoulder joint and the lateral chest wall drain into the axillary vain. As it crosses the first rib, the axillary vein becomes the subclavian vein. The main tributary of the subclavian vein is the external jugular vein. The subclavian vein unites with the internal jugular vein behind the medial aspect of the clavicle to form the brachiocephalic vein, also known as the innominate vein. The right and left brachiocephalic veins merge to form the superior vena cava, which subsequently enters the right atrium (**Fig. 3**).

An important distinguishing feature of deep in comparison with superficial veins is that the deep

This work was not supported by any grant.
The author has nothing to disclose.
Portions of text adapted from Allan, McDicken, Pozniak, Dubbins. Clinical Doppler ultrasound, 3rd edition. Churchill Livingstone, in press; with permission.
Department of Radiology, University of Wisconsin School of Medicine and Public Health, E3/311 Clinical Science Center, 600 Highland Avenue, Madison, WI 53792-3252, USA
E-mail address: mpozniak@uwhealth.org

doi:10.1016/j.cult.2011.08.001
1556-858X/11/$ – see front matter © 2011 Elsevier Inc. All rights reserved.

Box 1
Factors increasing risk for UEDVT

Central venous catheterization

Strenuous upper extremity exercise or anatomic abnormalities causing venous compression

Inherited thrombophilia

Acquired hypercoagulable states including pregnancy, oral contraceptive use, and cancer

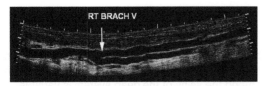

Fig. 1. Longitudinal extended composite view of the right brachial vein (RT BRACH V). Note the high extent of the duplication, almost to the axillary region (*arrow*).

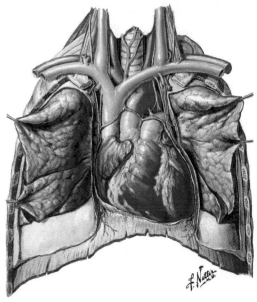

Fig. 3. Central venous anatomy of the upper thorax. Due to the close proximity to the right atrium, cardiac periodicity (ASVD waveform) should be routinely observed within these veins. (*From* netterimages.com, downloaded July 25, 2011, #833; with permission.)

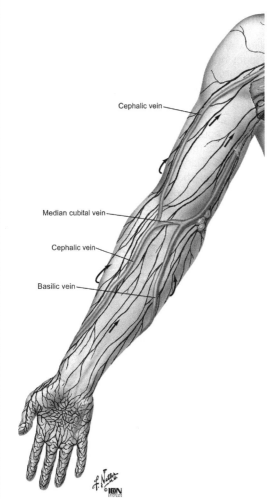

Fig. 2. Superficial venous anatomy of the upper extremity. (*From* netterimages.com, downloaded July 25, 2011, #4764; with permission.)

veins run parallel with their concomitant artery (**Fig. 4**A, B). The superficial veins course independently of the arterial system.

Perforating veins traverse between the deep and superficial system throughout the forearm and arm, forming important pathways of collateralization in the presence of partial thrombosis. In the absence of thrombus they are typically too small to see, but become more pronounced when they are recruited to divert flow around a clot (**Fig. 5**).

Valves are present within the veins of the UE. As one moves peripherally the location of the first valve is quite variable, but typically is encountered in the proximal brachial vein. Valve leaflets should be delicate and should move briskly with fluctuations in flow direction throughout the venous waveform. The sinus of the valve leaflets should be relatively free of echoes (**Fig. 6**).

SCANNING TECHNIQUE

The ultrasound examination of the UE veins for DVT relies on similar principles to examination of lower extremity venous examination: imaging, compression, and Doppler.

The study is typically performed with the patient in the supine position and the arm in a neutral anatomic position. The arm should be partially abducted to examine the axillary vein. If the arm is abducted completely, the axillary vein may become occluded as it crosses (and becomes compressed) between the clavicle and the first rib.

A linear transducer is used to perform the study. Seven to 12 MHz is a good frequency range to begin the study, as it provides sufficient penetration, particularly in large or edematous arms. A higher-frequency transducer may be used for superficial veins or in thinner arms. It is important to ensure that the Doppler settings are tuned for the slower velocities found in veins.

Standard venous compression is used throughout the arm and neck for the superficial and deep veins (**Fig. 7**). In the subclavian and central veins, however, this diagnostic tool cannot be applied.

Thrombus may be directly visualized in the vein lumen. Thrombus appears as echogenic material affixed to the vessel wall. The normal UE veins are easily compressible, but a clot will prevent the apposition of the walls of the vein. Light transducer pressure will obliterate the lumen of the normal vein and effectively rule out the presence of a clot. Compression should be light because fresh thrombus is soft and gelatinous. Firm pressure can produce a degree of compression, which may give a false impression of patency. Compression should be performed in the transverse plane, because if it is done in the longitudinal plane a thrombosed vein may disappear as it moves out of the scan plane, rather than because it has been compressed. A further reason for scanning in the transverse plane is that duplicated veins will be identified more reliably.

Color Doppler is a useful adjunct to confirm venous patency. A widely patent vein should fully saturate with color (**Fig. 8**). The color Doppler signal in the larger central veins normally fluctuates in direction. As a result of right atrial contraction the a-wave pushes back on venous return, resulting in a temporary reversal of flow. If an image is frozen during the brief moment of the a-wave, it is best not to archive that image because it may lead to suspicion of flow reversal by an uninformed viewer of the study.

With slow flow or poorly distended veins, one can enhance the perception of the color signal by asking the patient to perform a Valsalva maneuver. The resultant increased intrathoracic pressure resists venous return and allows more blood to pool peripherally. Subsequently, the patient is asked to exhale and clench his or her fist. Manual compression may also be applied to the forearm, but usually requires an assistant. The squeeze should be rapid and firm to propel blood up the veins. This action forces additional blood return in the venous system, enhancing the perceived

Doppler signal. In the larger veins with the color Doppler pulse repetition frequency set relatively low, with a brisk augment, aliasing may occur (**Fig. 9**); this should be recognized as a Doppler artifact. With the pulse repetition frequency adjusted to a higher level, the wall filter may suppress perception of slower laminar flow along the wall (**Fig. 10**). This appearance too can be confusing; care must be taken to not misinterpret this artifact as a clot adherent to the wall.

The UE spectral Doppler flow profile can be used to great diagnostic advantage. Because the veins of the UE are in close proximity to the heart, it is normal to see brisk cardiac periodicity in the Doppler flow profile. This characteristic tracing (atherosclerotic vascular disease [ASVD]) is quite complex (**Fig. 11**). The presence of this periodicity is a reassuring finding that is best seen when there is a wide-open conduit between the point of Doppler interrogation and the right atrium. Its absence indicates the presence of thrombus in the central veins, which normally cannot be imaged because of overlying lung and bone.

UPPER LIMB AND JUGULAR VEIN THROMBOSIS

The same principles used in lower extremity DVT studies apply to examination of the upper limb and neck veins. Lack of compressibility of the deep veins of the arm and neck and/or absence of flow on color or power Doppler are diagnostic of thrombosis (**Fig. 12**). The larger, more proximal veins, such as the axillary and subclavian, cannot be compressed, due to their location; diagnosis of thrombosis in these vessels will therefore depend on careful assessment using Doppler. Indirect signs of thrombosis include loss of respiratory phasicity or cardiac periodicity, which indicates proximal occlusion; such signs are useful if central vein (innominate or superior vena cava) thrombosis is suspected. Respiratory phasicity and cardiac periodicity can be modified by asking the patient to breathe deeply, hold his or her breath, or perform a Valsalva maneuver. After the release of Valsalva, absence of a surge in antegrade flow indicates a central clot. Comparison with flow dynamics on the contralateral side may be helpful in localizing the level of the clot.

DIAGNOSIS OF DVT

The lumen of a normal vein is anechoic and, on color Doppler, the entire lumen should fill with color, particularly with augmentation of flow. Thrombus fills the vein lumen with nonmobile echogenic material (**Fig. 13**). Color Doppler reveals

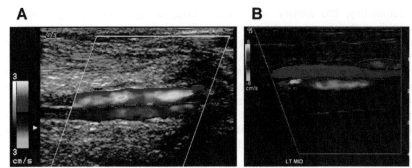

Fig. 4. (*A*) Longitudinal view of the left brachial artery and vein. The fact that the artery and vein course together defines them as part of the deep venous system. (*B*) Longitudinal view of the mid arm. Brachial artery in a different patient with paired adjacent veins. Venous duplication is a pitfall for the diagnosis of thrombosis. Finding one compressible vein near an artery may mask the presence of thrombus within the second vein.

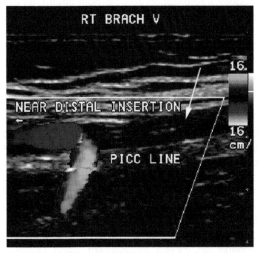

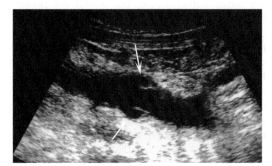

Fig. 6. Normal venous valves. Note the delicate thin leaflets, in an open position at this phase of flow. Note the anechoic cusps behind the valves, free of thrombus (*arrows*).

Fig. 5. A peripherally inserted central catheter (PICC) line is present in this brachial vein, partially occluded by thrombus (*arrow*). An enlarged perforating vein (*blue*) communicates to this brachial vein reestablishing flow above the level of the clot (*red*).

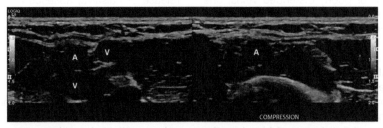

Fig. 7. Transverse view of the arm at the level just below the axilla. The brachial and basilic veins (V) are widely patent on the noncompressed view on the left. On the right, after compression, only the artery (A) is visible. The veins have been compressed to the point of occlusion, which effectively rules out the presence of thrombus.

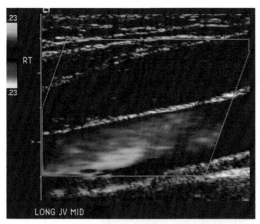

Fig. 8. Longitudinal view of the jugular vein. Color fully saturates the lumen of this vessel, effectively ruling out the presence of thrombus.

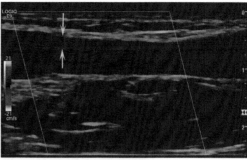

Fig. 10. Color Doppler image of a brachial vein with the pulse repetition frequency set for high-velocity flow. Note that color saturates only the central higher-velocity lamina in the middle of this vessel. No color saturation is seen along the wall (*arrows*); this is an artifact and should not be confused with mural thrombus.

a flow void in the affected area (**Fig. 14**). Although fresh thrombus is relatively hypoechoic, it becomes increasingly echogenic as it matures. In addition, fresh thrombus has a tendency to expand the vein and make it look rounder and fuller than a normal vessel.[2]

Fresh thrombus is not particularly adherent to the vein wall, so that flow may be seen around the periphery of the clot on color Doppler (see **Fig. 14**). Older thrombus becomes increasingly echogenic, adherent to the vein wall, and contracts as it becomes more organized and fibrotic, which may result in the vein being reduced to a relatively small echoic structure that may be difficult to identify. More commonly the thrombus may retract to one side of the vein, resulting in an asymmetric lumen on color Doppler. In patients with chronic reoccurring thrombosis a new clot may develop over an older clot, and an irregular mix of echotexture may be seen occupying the vein lumen (**Fig. 15**).

Normally flowing blood is anechoic. Individual red blood cells (RBCs) are too small to reflect the incoming sound wave. However, RBCs in certain conditions may stick to each other. These stacks of RBCs are called Rouleaux (**Fig. 16**). Conditions that cause rouleau formation include infections, multiple myeloma, inflammatory and connective tissue disorders, diabetes mellitus, cancers, and pregnancy. These stacks of red cells become a large enough target to interact with the insonating beam and therefore manifest as echoes in the

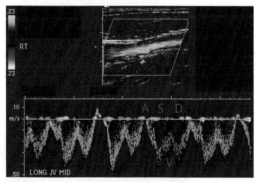

Fig. 11. Spectral Doppler tracing of the jugular vein. Cardiac periodicity corresponding to the right atrial activity is manifest on this tracing. With atrial contraction, a brief reverse component of flow is present known, as the A wave, subsequently followed by rapid antegrade flow into the empty right atrium. On saturation, the slowing of antegrade rate flow is known as the S wave. Then the tricuspid valve opens and antegrade velocity surges to fill the empty right ventricle; this is known as the D wave. Subsequently antegrade flow slows again as the ventricle becomes saturated: the D wave. Visualization of this waveform effectively guarantees patency of the venous system between the right atrium and the point of interrogation.

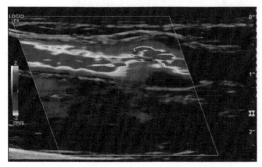

Fig. 9. Longitudinal view of the brachial vein with color Doppler settings at a very sensitive level. Note the color shift in the center of the vessel; this is caused by aliasing and should not be confused with flow reversal.

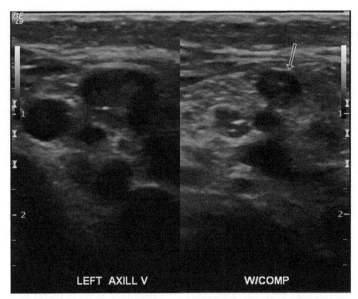

Fig. 12. Transverse view of the vessels near the left axilla. The noncompressed view of the axillary vein shows some echogenic material within it. On compression (*arrow*), the walls cannot be brought together, due to the clot. Because this is a relatively fresh clot, however, it can be partially compressed.

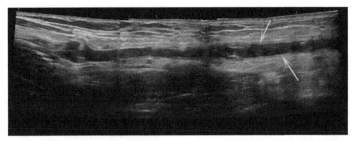

Fig. 13. Extended field-of-view image of the right basilic vein. Note the lumen, relatively distended, and filled with echogenic thrombus (*arrows*).

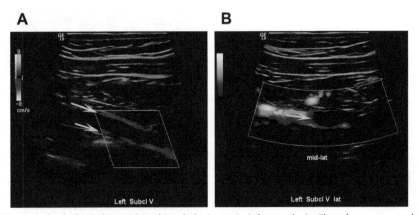

Fig. 14. (*A*) Relatively fresh thrombus within the subclavian vein is hypoechoic. Flow, however, can be seen along the periphery of the thrombus, between thrombus and vessel wall (*arrow*). This appearance is best appreciated with Valsalva release and an augmentation maneuver. (*B*) The leading edge of the thrombus is defined as this filling defect within the mid-subclavian vein (*arrow*). Note power Doppler manifesting color flow around the clot.

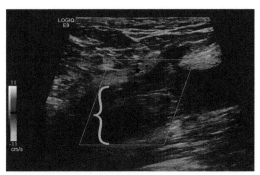

Fig. 15. Clot is present within this vein (*bracket*). Note the mixed echo texture, a function of a new clot superimposed on an old clot.

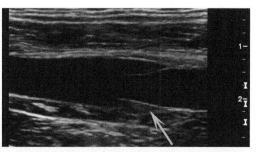

Fig. 17. Valve leaflets within a vein. Note the deeper valve leaflet has echogenic material behind it (*arrow*). On compression, this was easily dislodged. This appearance is a manifestation of rouleau formation in an area of slow sluggish flow.

bloodstream. Such stacks are more likely to occur in areas where flow is slow, especially in the sinus behind the cusps of valves (**Fig. 17**). If compression on a valve easily dislodges these Rouleaux aggregates, this is nothing more than rouleau formation. If, however, the echogenic material remains lodged after adequate compression, early clot formation is diagnosed (**Fig. 18**).

SPECTRAL DOPPLER FINDINGS
Spontaneous Flow and Respiratory Variation

If there is thrombus occluding the vein, there will not be any flow detected in the lumen at the level of the thrombus. Patent segments below the thrombus may show some slow antegrade flow, particularly if collateral channels are adequate, but they will

not show any respiratory variation, and the augmentation response is damped (**Fig. 19**).

Augmentation

Normal venous flow is slow. Its perception on Doppler can be improved by compression distal to the point of assessment (**Fig. 20**). In a normal venous system there will be a rapid rise and fall in the frequency shift, whereas if there is a thrombosed venous segment it will resist flow with damping, or absence, of the augmentation response (**Fig. 21**). The squeeze should not be violent or excessive, as patients will often be tender; in addition there is a small potential risk of dislodging a fresh friable thrombus, producing a pulmonary embolus. The risk of this is small, and reports of this type of event are few.[3]

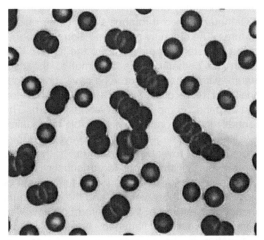

Fig. 16. Micrograph of red blood cells. Note that several stacks of red blood cells clump together in the shape of a roll of lifesavers. When clustered they can reflect the incoming sound wave, causing visualization of nonthrombosed blood (original magnification ×30).

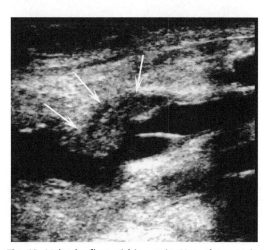

Fig. 18. Valve leaflets within a vein. Note the anterior leaflet has echogenic material behind it as well as extending beyond the cusp (*arrows*). Compression was unable to dislodge this. This material is early thrombus beginning to form behind the cusp of a valve and propagating downstream.

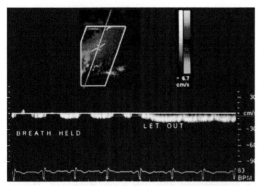

Fig. 19. Spectral Doppler tracing of a distended vein shows relatively little flow during breath-hold with Valsalva. On release (let out), however, there is very little surge in antegrade velocity, which speaks in favor of a central thrombus. Note also that there is no cardiac periodicity in this large central vein: another clue.

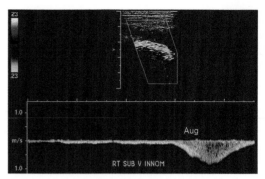

Fig. 21. Spectral Doppler imaging of this right subclavian vein approximating the innominate vein. Although fully distended, at rest there is no periodicity and very slow flow. On augmentation (Aug) there is a feeble response, which helps confirm the presence of a central thrombus.

Flow in Collateral Channels

When the normal venous channels are occluded, blood may be seen in collateral veins. In the acute stage intramuscular channels will not have developed significantly, but increased velocity and flow may be seen. Over a period of several weeks the intramuscular venous channels will expand and may become apparent on color Doppler (see **Fig. 5**). Therefore, their visualization suggests chronic thrombosis.

Collateral perforating veins themselves may serve as a pathway for the propagation of a clot from the superficial to the deep system (**Fig. 22**). This aspect is important in the diagnosis of thrombophlebitis. Deep thrombophlebitis carries a worse prognosis and requires more aggressive therapy.

Chronic Changes After DVT

Normal valves may be seen moving gently in the currents from blood passing them, particularly in the larger veins (see **Fig. 6**). If valve cusps appear rigid or fixed, this usually represents the sequela of prior DVT.

The walls of a normal vein are smooth and unobtrusive. Following recanalization after DVT they become irregular, thickened, and echogenic. Rarely, calcification may develop.

Catheter-related thrombosis has some unique features. The clot may propagate along the length of the catheter or it may cling to the tip (**Fig. 23**). When the catheter tip is proximal to the right atrium, within the superior vena cava, brachiocephalic, or more distal veins, a clot may develop and expand, compromising venous return. The centrally located ones are impossible to visualize by ultrasound imaging alone; however, Doppler findings may reveal its presence. If the large central veins of the upper torso (subclavian and jugular) are markedly distended, a full column of blood between those vessels and the right atrium should transmit the ASVD waveform. If, however, Doppler reveals a flattened flow profile, an obstruction to the antegrade flow of blood and the retrograde propagation of the waveform infers the presence of a central clot (**Fig. 24**). If these findings are in both right and left subclavian and jugular veins, the level of obstruction is at the

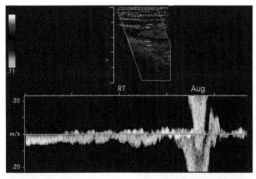

Fig. 20. Longitudinal view of a normal right brachial vein. The spectral Doppler tracing shows relatively uniform flow, presumably due to intervening valves between the point of interrogation and the right atrium. However, with a brisk augment (Aug) there is a rapid increase in velocity to the point of causing aliasing; this is a normal finding. In an arm that is at rest the venous flow can be very slow. Another tool to increase venous flow is to have the patient exercise the forearm by repeatedly clenching a towel or pumping his or her fist. This action increases metabolism, thereby increasing arterial inflow and venous outflow.

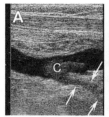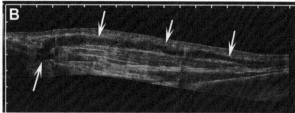

Fig. 22. (A) Echogenic thrombus is seen in a perforating vein (*arrows*). As this vein enters a larger deeper vein, a clot (C) is seen extending out, compromising flow within the lumen of the larger vessel. (B) Extended composite view of the cephalic vein shows it filled with echogenic thrombus (*downward arrows*). At the cephalad aspect it is seen diving deep, with thrombus extending into the axillary vein (*upward arrow*). This was a palpable tender cord with the clinical diagnosis of superficial thrombophlebitis. The fact that the infected clot entered the deep venous system complicates therapy.

inferior vena cava. If only one side manifests these changes, the obstructing clot is inferred to be at the level of that brachiocephalic vein.

Clinical Significance

Baarslag and colleagues[4] compared ultrasound Doppler with venography for the diagnosis of upper limb DVT and found 82% sensitivity and 82% specificity. These investigators reported that 63% of patients who had thrombosis had associated malignant disease, and 14% of patients who had thrombosis had an indwelling central venous catheter but without malignant disease.

The risk of clinically significant pulmonary embolus from upper limb DVT is relatively low compared with lower limb DVT, but the reported frequency of occurrence varies widely. Mustafa

and colleagues[5] reported a series of 65 patients with arm vein thrombosis, none of whom were found to have symptomatic pulmonary emboli.

Bernardi and colleagues[6] stated that UEDVT accounts for about 10% of all episodes of venous thrombosis. Although risk factors are well defined, in their patient cohort 20% of episodes of UEDVT were unexplained. Bernardi and colleagues stated that up to one-third of the patients with UEDVT may develop pulmonary embolism, and emphasized that UEDVT should no longer be considered a rare and benign condition.

By contrast, Kommareddy and colleagues[7] reported that UEDVT only makes up approximately 1% to 4% of all episodes of DVT. These investigators did emphasize that unexplained or recurrent UEDVT should prompt a vigorous search for coagulation disorders or underlying malignancy.

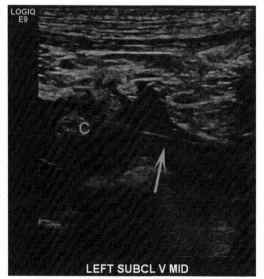

Fig. 23. A catheter is identified in the left subclavian vein (*arrow*). At its tip is a large echogenic clump of thrombus (C) adherent to the catheter tip.

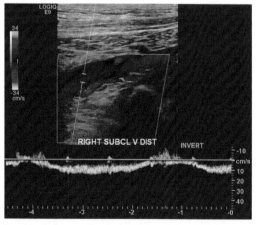

Fig. 24. Color and spectral Doppler imaging of the right subclavian vein. Flow is passing centrally, but spectral Doppler shows it to be relatively slow and there is no periodicity. Only respiratory variation is perceived and it actually manifests flow reversal. This appearance indicates a central thrombus at the level of either the right innominate or inferior vena cava.

Levy and colleagues[8] reported that the incidence of pulmonary embolism attributed to previously documented UEDVT is relatively small (around 1%). Anticoagulation therapy is best suited to treat the symptoms of UEDVT but does relatively little to reduce the risk of pulmonary embolism. Because patients with UEDVT are typically very ill, the associated risks of therapeutic anticoagulation must be carefully weighed.

Hingorani and colleagues,[9] however, followed a large cohort of patients with diagnosed UEDVT, and found an overall mortality rate in these patients approaching 30%. Of this cohort, however, only 5% developed pulmonary emboli. Mortality in the majority of these individuals was from coincident morbidities, more likely responsible than the pulmonary embolism for their demise. Therefore, the high association mortality of UEDVT may be due to the underlying characteristics of the patient's disease process and may not be a direct consequence of the UEDVT itself.

SUMMARY

Ultrasonography is a safe and reliable method for assessing the possibility of UEDVT in symptomatic patients. The oncology patient with arm swelling and an indwelling catheter is the perfect candidate for this study. The exact risk of life-threatening pulmonary embolism in these individuals is yet to be defined with certainty.

REFERENCES

1. Baxter GM. The role of ultrasound in deep vein thrombosis [editorial]. Clin Radiol 1997;52:1–3.
2. Hertzberg BS, Kliewer MA, DeLong DM, et al. Sonographic assessment of lower limb vein diameters: implications for the diagnosis and characterization of deep venous thrombosis. Am J Roentgenol 1997; 168:1253–7.
3. Perlin SJ. Pulmonary embolism during compression US of the lower extremity. Radiology 1992;184:165–6.
4. Baarslag HJ, van Beek EJ, Koopman MM, et al. Prospective study of color duplex ultrasonography compared with contrast venography in patients suspected of having deep venous thrombosis of the upper extremities. Ann Intern Med 2002;136:865–72.
5. Mustafa S, Stein PD, Patel KC, et al. Upper extremity deep venous thrombosis. Chest 2003;123:1953–6.
6. Bernardi E, Pesavento R, Prandoni P. Upper extremity deep venous thrombosis. Semin Thromb Hemost 2006;32(7):729–36.
7. Kommareddy A, Zaroukian MH, Hassouna HI. Upper extremity deep venous thrombosis. Semin Thromb Hemost 2002;28(1):89–99.
8. Levy MM, Bach C, Fisher-Snowden R, et al. Upper extremity deep venous thrombosis: reassessing the risk for subsequent pulmonary embolism. Ann Vasc Surg 2011;25(4):442–7.
9. Hingorani A, Ascher E, Markevich N, et al. Risk factors for mortality in patients with upper extremity and internal jugular deep venous thrombosis. J Vasc Surg 2005;41(3):476–8.

Ultrasound Evaluation of Carotid Intima Media Thickness: The Hows and Whys

Igor Latich, MD*, Leslie M. Scoutt, MD

KEYWORDS

- Ultrasound • Cardiovascular disease
- Carotid intima media • Atherogenesis

An estimated 17.1 million people died of cardiovascular disease (CVD) in 2004, representing 29% of all global deaths.[1,2] Of these deaths, nearly 7.2 million were caused by coronary artery disease (CAD) and 5.7 million were caused by stroke. Mortality statistics reported by the World Health Organization indicated that CVD was the underlying cause of death in 37.3% of all deaths in the United States in 2003 and that 32% of all deaths from CVD occurred prematurely or before the age of 75 years (close to the average life expectancy in the United States).[1,2] Atherosclerosis is well recognized as the pathologic cause of most cardiovascular events.[3] Because atherosclerosis begins early in life and can progress silently for decades, there has been great interest in identifying asymptomatic high-risk individuals before an acute, and sometimes fatal, event occurs.[1,4] Smoking, hypertension, and diabetes, as well as increased plasma levels of fibrinogen, low-density lipoprotein (LDL), and cholesterol are some of the widely accepted risk factors for the development of atherosclerosis and CVD.[5,6] However, these risk factors do not necessarily reflect the presence or extent of the atherosclerotic process at the level of the arterial wall.[7] Nor can these risk factors be used to measure either progression of atherosclerosis or response to therapy.[7] However, changes in carotid intima media thickness (CIMT) have been found to correlate well with changes in atherosclerotic burden.[8] In addition, increased thickness of the intima media layer has been shown in several prospective multicenter studies to be an independent risk factor for asymptomatic CVD, myocardial infarction, and stroke.[5,7,9–14] Hence, measurement of CIMT with B-mode ultrasound (US) has been proposed as a noninvasive, sensitive technique for identifying and quantifying subclinical vascular disease and for evaluating CVD risk.[14] This article reviews the basic pathophysiology of atherogenesis, the data supporting the role of CIMT as a surrogate marker for cardiovascular disease, and the current controversies regarding the methodology for optimal measurement of the CIMT.

ATHEROGENESIS

On the microscopic level, hyperlipidemia is one of the primary initiating events in the development of atherosclerosis. Oxidization of LDL that has infiltrated into the intima of the arterial wall is believed to trigger an inflammatory response resulting in endothelial dysfunction manifested by the release of substances that promote adherence of platelets, monocytes, and lymphocytes to the endothelial surface and ultimately the migration of leukocytes into the subendothelial space.[15–20] Within the subendothelial space, monocytes differentiate into inflammatory cells, including macrophages, which take up or phagocytize the LDL located within the intima via scavenger and toll-like receptors.[21–23] Cholesterol and LDL that cannot be mobilized and destroyed by the

Department of Diagnostic Radiology, Yale University School of Medicine, 333 Cedar Street, PO Box 208042, New Haven, CT 06520-8042, USA
* Corresponding author.
E-mail address: igor.latic@yale.edu

Ultrasound Clin 6 (2011) 445–461
doi:10.1016/j.cult.2011.08.002
1556-858X/11/$ – see front matter © 2011 Elsevier Inc. All rights reserved.

monocyte accumulate within the cell's cytoplasm in the form of cytosolic droplets, ultimately transforming the macrophage into a foam cell that is the prototypical cell of an atherosclerotic plaque.[17,21,24] In addition, the toll-like receptors seem to initiate a further cascade of inflammatory response involving inflammatory cytokines, chemokines, proteases, and free radicals.[24,25] Mast cells and T-cell infiltrates are always present in atherosclerotic lesions, which provides further confirmation of the importance of inflammation in atherogenesis.[24] Ultimately, the balance between inflammatory and antiinflammatory activity is believed to determine the rate of progression of an atherosclerotic plaque.[24] Infection with *Chlamydia* and cytomegalovirus (CMV) may also affect the progression of atherosclerosis; CMV infection or colonization seems to be especially important in the development of atherosclerosis, which may be extremely aggressive, in patients after transplantation.[26–28]

As atherosclerosis progresses and reactive physiologic compensation causes thickening of the intima media complex of the arterial wall, the oxygen diffusion threshold is exceeded, inducing hypoxia and ischemia, which triggers the release of a cascade of inflammatory growth factors that results in neovascularization of plaque and proliferation of the vasa vasorum within the adventitia, which is a histologic hallmark of symptomatic atherosclerosis.[29] In addition, the inflammatory

response stimulates the migration and proliferation of smooth muscle cells within the plaque.[30] Wall thickening may occur in the intimal layer or in the muscular, medial layer (**Figs. 1** and **2**). However, the muscular media layer is thin in the carotid artery. Hence, thickening of the arterial wall of the carotid artery is essentially caused by intimal thickening.[31]

On the macroscopic level, atherosclerotic plaques are composed of 3 cell types (endothelial, smooth muscle, and inflammatory cells), connective tissue elements, lipids, and debris, all of which primarily accumulate within the intima of the arterial wall.[31] Foam cells and lipid droplets form a central core that is covered by a cap of smooth muscle cells and a collagen-rich matrix of connective tissue. Neovascularity is commonly observed within plaque itself. In addition, the vasa vasorum proliferates within the outer adventitial layer of the vessel wall underneath the plaque, particularly inflammatory plaque. Intraplaque hemorrhage may or may not be present. Atheromas typically grow at the shoulder regions where inflammatory cells such as T cells, mast cells, and macrophages are most abundant.[32–34] Atherosclerosis and plaque most commonly develop in areas of turbulent flow with high sheer stress, such as arterial bifurcations.

In response to plaque deposition and thickening of the vessel wall, the vessel initially expands outwards to accommodate the growing plaque. This process is termed positive remodeling.

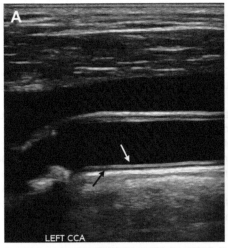 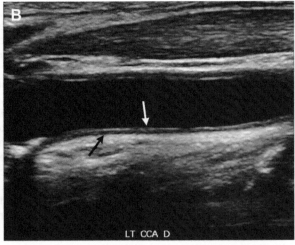

Fig. 1. (*A, B*) Normal carotid intima media layer. Sagittal gray-scale US images from 2 different patients of the common carotid artery showing the normal intima media layer seen to best advantage in the far wall of the vessel. The more superficial echogenic line (*white arrows*) represents the intima and the interface of the intima with the vessel lumen. Immediately underneath is a hypoechoic layer (*black arrows*), which represents the media layer of the vessel wall. The underlying echogenic linear layer represents the adventitia and the interface with the surrounding soft tissues.

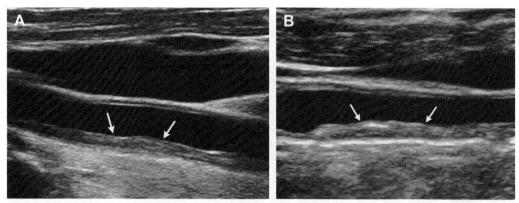

Fig. 2. (*A, B*) Thickened carotid intima media layer. Sagittal gray-scale US images from 2 different patients showing thickening of the carotid intima media layers (*arrows*) seen to best advantage involving the far wall of the common carotid artery. In addition to the thickening, note heterogeneity of the echotexture of the wall and loss of the normal striated echopattern described in **Fig. 1.**

Positive remodeling results in widening of the vessel diameter without significant narrowing of the lumen. Hence, there may be extensive plaque burden with minimal narrowing of the residual lumen. Nonetheless, such large plaques have been shown to be significantly associated with acute coronary syndromes despite the absence of luminal stenosis.[35] It is thought that plaque rupture and/or endothelial erosion of such large, activated plaques expose thrombogenic elements within the plaque core, such as phospholipids, tissue factors, and platelet adhesive molecules, to the blood stream, resulting in the formation of thrombus on the surface of the plaque, and that many clinically important cardiovascular events are caused by distal infarction from embolization of intraluminal thrombus on the surface of such activated plaques.[30,36,37] In addition, activated macrophages within the plaque also release proteinases and proteolytic enzymes that can lead to intraplaque hemorrhage from the vasa vasorum, or plaque neovascularity and consequent swelling of the plaque, which is believed to precipitate rupture of the plaque surface.[30] Eventually, positive remodeling will not be able to accommodate continued growth of the plaque, and, in advanced stages of the disease, encroachment into the vessel lumen occurs, creating a luminal stenosis.[38] Thrombus that develops on the surface of plaque where the lumen is significantly narrowed is particularly unstable because the kinetic energy from the increased velocity and the turbulence of blood flow at the site of the stenosis increases the risk of distal embolization.

Much research has been focused on the prospective identification of such vulnerable or activated plaque, which is characterized microscopically by an increased number of inflammatory cells (activated macrophages and T-lymphocytes), neovascularity, and thinning or rupture of the fibrous cap. Most of these features cannot be directly visualized using current imaging techniques. However, intraplaque hemorrhage, whether from rupture of the capsule or disruption of the vasa vasorum and vessels within the plaque, can sometimes be visualized on high-resolution ultrasound (US) or magnetic resonance (MR) images. On US, hemorrhagic plaque is typically hypoechoic or sometimes even anechoic as well as heterogeneous (**Fig. 3**). Homogeneous or echogenic plaque (**Fig. 4**) is more likely to be stable.[39–41] Several prospective studies have shown that heterogeneous plaque with focal hypoechoic/anechoic areas or plaque with irregular surface characteristics is associated with increased risk of neurologic events.[42–44] However, there is significant interobserver and intraobserver variability reported in the assessment and/or identification of hypoechoic plaque. In addition, fibrous plaque and lipid-laden plaque also may appear hypoechoic. Hence, hypoechoic plaque is a nonspecific US finding. Thus, the role of gray-scale US in identifying vulnerable plaque is generally considered limited. Recently, several studies postulated that the detection of increased plaque neovascularity using intravenous contrast enhancement on US may serve as a marker for vulnerable plaque (see later discussion).

SCREENING FOR ATHEROSCLEROSIS USING IMAGING

Narrowing of the coronary arteries as measured on angiography is predictive of coronary events.[7]

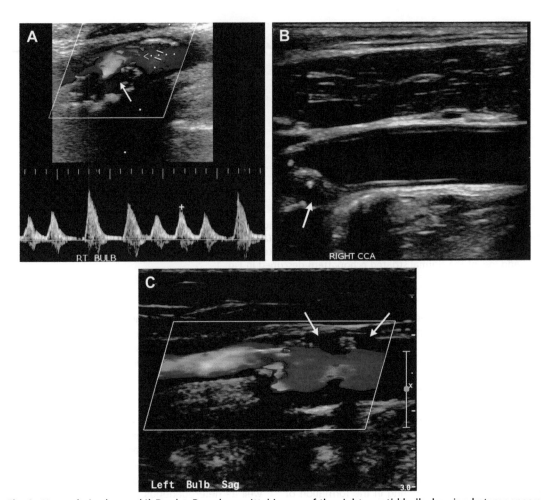

Fig. 3. Hypoechoic plaque. (*A*) Duplex Doppler sagittal image of the right carotid bulb showing heterogeneous plaque with a focal hypoechoic area (*arrow*). (*B*) Sagittal gray-scale image of the distal right common carotid artery and bulb in a second patient showing heterogeneous plaque with punctuate brightly echogenic foci, possibly representing calcification as well as a focal hypoechoic area (*arrow*). (*C*) Color Doppler sagittal image of the left carotid bulb in a third patient showing heterogeneous plaque along the near wall with 2 discrete focal hypoechoic areas (*arrows*). Hypoechoic plaque, particularly if focal within heterogeneous plaque, suggests intraplaque hemorrhage. However, this finding is nonspecific and is seen with fibrous fatty plaque as well.

However, the early phase of atherosclerosis when atheromas do not protrude into the vessel lumen cannot be documented on conventional or digital angiograms because only the vessel lumen, and not the vessel wall itself, is visualized.[7] Hence, angiography alone routinely underestimates disease burden, as studies comparing postmortem histology with angiographic measurements have shown.[45] In addition, coronary angiography is invasive, expensive, and exposes the patient to the risks associated with ionizing radiation and the administration of iodinated intravenous contrast. Thus, the use of coronary angiography as a screening strategy in asymptomatic patients is not feasible, and there is much

interest in the potential of noninvasive imaging techniques such as MR imaging, cardiac computed tomography (CT), computed tomographic angiography (CTA), and US for the detection of asymptomatic atherosclerosis as well as for evaluation of progression of the disease.[46]

Measurement of CIMT has been proposed as a surrogate marker for the presence of coronary atherosclerosis.[7] The American Heart Association currently recommends that the CIMT be measured to assess risk for atherosclerosis and CVD.[47] CIMT evaluation with US is noninvasive, inexpensive, and does not expose patients to the risks associated with the use of ionizing radiation or intravenous iodinated contrast. Furthermore,

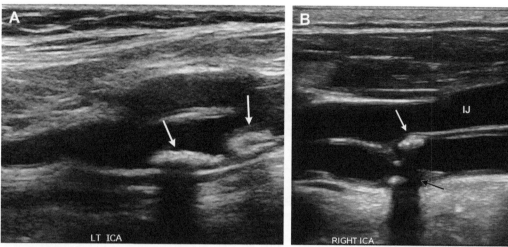

Fig. 4. Echogenic plaque (*A*) Note 2 highly echogenic plaques (*arrows*) on this sagittal gray-scale image of the origin of the left internal carotid artery (ICA). Distal shadowing is noted below the more superior plaque. (*B*) Note multiple foci of echogenic plaque at the origin of the right ICA on this sagittal gray-scale image of a second patient. The apparent focal area of hypoechoic plaque along the far wall (*black arrow*) is artifact from shadowing from the more anterior plaque (*white arrow*). Echogenic plaque has been reported to have no prognostic significance in most studies and does not necessarily indicate calcification, although calcification is more likely if shadowing is observed. IJ, internal jugular vein.

measurement of CIMT has the potential to identify atherosclerosis in the vessel wall before narrowing of the lumen develops. On longitudinal images of the carotid artery, the CIMT is measured from the echogenic interface of the intima with the anechoic vessel lumen to the echogenic adventitia. The hypoechoic media between these 2 parallel echogenic lines is included in the measurement (**Fig. 5**). Recent advances in equipment and measuring techniques, including edge-detection software (**Fig. 6**), have been reported to be associated with high interobserver and intra-observer reproducibility, at least in well-controlled research settings, making serial CIMT measurements a feasible method for monitoring changes in atherosclerosis with time and/or in response to therapeutic intervention.[48–51]

SUPPORTING DATA FOR THE ROLE OF CIMT AS A MARKER FOR CARDIOVASCULAR DISEASE

In 1986, Pignoli and colleagues[52] first reported a correlation between aortic wall thickness and atherosclerosis. Since that time, numerous large clinical trials have shown that CIMT significantly predicts future clinical cardiovascular events.[5,9,11,13,14,53,54] The Cardiovascular Health Study of 4476 patients more than 65 years of age and followed for 6 years reported in 1999 by O'Leary and colleagues[11] showed that the age-adjusted and sex-adjusted relative risk for

myocardial infarction (MI) and stroke was proportional to CIMT. In this study, the rate of stroke and MI in the highest quintile of CIMT was greater than 25% in comparison with less than 5% in the lowest quintile, yielding a risk in the highest quintile 3.87 times the risk in the lowest quintile.[11] The Atherosclerosis Risk in Communities Study published in 1997 by Chambliss and colleagues[5] studied more than 15,000 patients and also showed that increased CIMT was associated with increased risk of symptomatic CAD and stroke. Similar findings were reported in the Rotterdam Study.[53] A meta-analysis of 8 studies published in 2007 by Lorenz and colleagues[12] reaffirmed that increased CIMT was a strong predictor of future cardiovascular events. Specifically, an increase in CIMT by 0.1 mm increased the future risk of stroke by 13% to 18% and increased the risk of MI by 10% to 15%.[12] In a recent review of 33 studies, 29 showed a positive relationship between CIMT and CAD, with correlations ranging between 0.12 and 0.51.[54] Others have attempted to correlate CIMT values with the number of coronary arteries involved with atherosclerosis. Atherosclerosis of a single coronary artery in patients older than 65 years was associated with a CIMT of approx 0.9 mm, 2-vessel disease with a CIMT of 1.2 mm, and 3-vessel disease with a CIMT of 1.3 mm.[55]

Moreover, CIMT measurement has been shown to be an independent risk factor, as well as an equally strong predictor of cardiovascular events

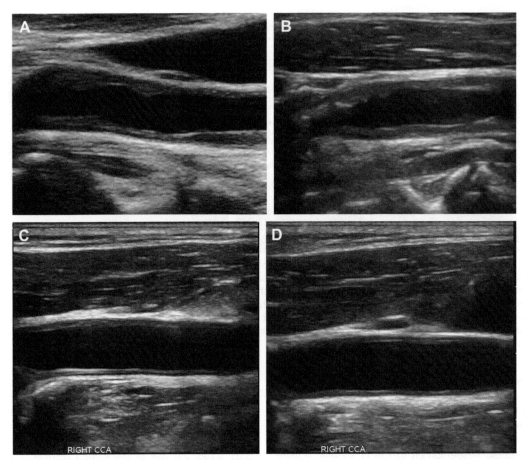

Fig. 5. Evaluation of the near wall of the carotid intima media layer. (*A, B*) In these 2 patients, the carotid intima media layer is substantially thicker and more irregular in the near (anterior) wall. Whether or not both the anterior and posterior walls should be measured and, if measured, whether or not the CIMT thickness should be reported separately, averaged, or a maximum measurement reported has not clearly been defined. Similarly, studies have not reported consensus on whether or not both the right and left CIMT should be evaluated. (*C, D*) Although some investigators have stated that the CIMT is usually thicker in the near (anterior) wall than in the far (posterior) wall, most researchers report that the CIMT is not as clearly visualized in the near wall because of near-field artifact as is seen in these 2 patients. Therefore, most investigators, including the ASE, recommend measuring the CIMT from the far wall.

as the traditionally described risk factors such as age, race, diabetes, cholesterol, hypertension, and smoking.[5,11,49] An increase of 1 standard deviation (SD) in combined intima media thickness was associated with a relative risk of 1.36 for MI or stroke. In contrast, an increase in age of 1 SD (5.5 years) was associated with a relative risk of 1.34, and an increase in systolic blood pressure of 1 SD (21.5 mm Hg) with a relative risk of 1.21.

Not only is increased CIMT an independent risk factor for CVD, but increased CIMT may be the only identifiable risk factor in some patients, and, therefore, may help to identify CVD in asymptomatic individuals without traditional risk factors. A study reported by Khot and colleagues[6] in 2003

examined the prevalence of 4 conventional CVD risk factors (smoking, diabetes, hypertension, and hyperlipidemia) in more than 120,000 patients who participated in cardiovascular clinical trials. Their data showed that approximately 15% of women and 19% of men did not have a single conventional risk factor.[6] Moreover, the number of patients with CVD without any of the 4 risk factors increased with age and exceeded 20% in women older than 75 years and in men older than 65 years.[6] Thus, CVD risk assessment with CIMT has particular relevance in the elderly, in whom borderline increase of multiple risk factors is common.[11] Furthermore, the association between traditional risk factors and CVD has

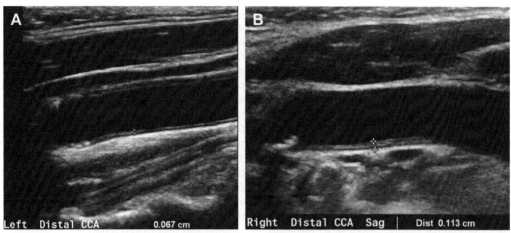

Fig. 6. Measurement of carotid intima media thickness with hand-placed calipers. (*A*) Sagittal gray-scale image of the distal left common carotid artery showing measurement of the normal CIMT. Measurement is typically made from the far or posterior wall approximately 1 cm from the carotid bulb. The vessel should be as parallel as possible to the surface of the transducer. Calipers with a + configuration should be used with the crosshair placed on the echogenic intima at the interface of the intima with the anechoic vessel lumen and at the echogenic interface of the adventitia with the hypoechoic media. In this patient, the CIMT measures 0.67 mm. (*B*) Sagittal gray-scale image of the distal right common carotid artery in a second patient showing increased CIMT, measuring 1.13 mm.

been shown to weaken in the later years of life, making it difficult to identify older patients with subclinical cardiovascular disease from traditional risk factors alone.[56,57]

A smaller study of 118 young patients (35–59 years) with 1 cardiovascular risk factor but no evidence of CVD found that 13% had CIMT greater than the 75th percentile (considered high risk), suggesting that even young people with seemingly low risk can have significant but asymptomatic atherosclerotic disease.[58] Thus, the addition of CIMT measurement to cardiovascular risk stratification protocols may help identify asymptomatic younger individuals who would benefit from aggressive preventive measures.[47,59] Several other studies have suggested that CIMT measurement can be effectively used to modify the Framingham Risk Score and improve classification of CVD risk.[60,61]

The aforementioned body of evidence validating CIMT measurement as a predictive marker for CVD has led to its application as a surrogate end point to assess treatment efficacy for atherosclerosis, such as for antihypertensive drugs, niacin, statins, and other lipid-lowering drugs, as well as behavior modification. The potential for enhancing the process of drug development by providing an easily measurable end point several years in advance of data analysis from clinical end point trials is enormous.[9] One of the first studies that evaluated the effect of statins on progression of subclinical atherosclerosis showed that treatment with rosuvastatin (Crestor) not only halted

progression of atherosclerosis, but reversed CIMT by 0.0014 mm annually versus the 0.0131-mm increase for placebo-treated subjects.[57] As a result of this trial, rosuvastatin was the first statin to be granted an indication for slowing the progression of atherosclerosis by the US Food and Drug Administration. The initial ARBITER (Arterial Biology for the Investigation of the Treatment Effects of Reducing Cholesterol) trial and follow-up report showed that marked LDL reduction (<100 mg/dL) with statin therapy induced CIMT regression in a 13-month period.[52,62] A recent meta-analysis of 7 statin trials revealed a statistical link between progression of CIMT and incidence of cardiovascular events.[63]

CONTROVERSIES REGARDING CIMT MEASUREMENT

The media is a hypoechoic linear structure that provides excellent contrast between the linear echogenic intima-lumen interface and the echogenic adventitia of the outer arterial wall (see **Fig. 1**). Imaging with B-mode US perpendicular to the longitudinal axis of the vessel using a high-frequency, linear-array transducer provides clear visualization of the carotid intima media layers in most patients (see **Figs. 1** and **2**). However, routine monitoring of CIMT in clinical practice outside of the research setting has been hampered by lack of standardized protocols.[8]

The methodologies in the previously described large multi-institutional studies have been fairly inconsistent. Some investigators report the maximum measurement, others average multiple values, and others report a mean. In addition, a universally accepted risk stratification scale has not been established. Some studies divided patients into quintiles; other studies used quartiles; other researchers advocate using absolute numbers adjusted for age, sex, and ethnicity; other studies investigated growth rate.

There has been no clear agreement on which segment of the carotid artery to measure. Common carotid artery (CCA) measurements tend to be more consistent and reproducible because the vessel is large, superficial, and typically courses parallel to the skin surface and transducer. The internal carotid artery (ICA) generally runs obliquely to the skin surface and is usually not as straight as the CCA, making consistent measurement more difficult. In studies in which both the CCA and ICA have been measured, data have been inconsistent regarding which vessel has the strongest correlation of CIMT with cardiovascular events. Both far-wall and near-wall measurements have been used, as well as an average of the two.[4,50] Feinstein[29] suggest that imaging the near wall is advantageous because of its thickness and increased propensity for atherosclerosis (see **Fig. 5**). However, near-field artifact commonly obscures visualization of the near wall (see **Fig. 5**) and some researchers report that US routinely underestimates near-wall CIMT by 20%, is more challenging technically, is less reproducible, and does not appreciably improve risk prediction.[63–65] In addition, near-wall CIMT measurement is believed to be less accurate because the ultrasound beam travels from more echogenic to less echogenic layers at the adventitia-media and intima-lumen interfaces in the near wall.[66] Some studies advocate unilateral measurement and others require averaging of measurements of the CIMT from the right and left.

Controversy also exists as to whether it is accurate to measure CIMT with hand-placed calipers (see **Fig. 6**) or whether it is better to make an automated measurement using edge-detection software for a 1-cm length of the arterial wall (**Fig. 7**). Most now favor the use of automated measurement with manual override capabilities. However, automated measurements, although more reproducible, are generally wider than measurements made with hand-placed calipers. Thus, standardized charts derived from measurements made by calipers may not be valid for automated measurements.

Another frequently voiced concern with CIMT measurements is operator dependence. The sonographer must measure CIMT in fractions of a millimeter, which is at the limit of resolution for even the best US equipment (0.1–0.2 mm spatial resolution). Thus, measurement of such a small structure has enormous potential for significant percentile measurement error (**Fig. 8**). Interobserver variability as defined by Spearman correlation coefficients have been reported in the range of 0.75 to 0.86.[11] Intraobserver variability is also reportedly high, between 0.69 and 0.73 in one study.[9] This makes risk stratification challenging because differences between categories tend to be minute. For example, in one study, the individual quartiles varied by less than 0.1 mm and the difference between the highest and lowest quartile was less than 0.3 mm.[67]

The introduction of edge-detection software has reduced reader variation and improved reproducibility.[68] Using edge-detection or border-detection software, Gepner and colleagues[69] reported that readers (whether experienced or novice) were able to detect CIMT differences of 0.011 mm (±0.004 mm) and 0.022 mm (±0.004 mm), compared with CIMT measurements of the same images by a reference laboratory. Intraobserver reproducibility was high, with mean absolute differences of 0.003 mm and 0.040 mm for the experienced and novice readers, respectively.

Additional confounding factors that should be considered when interpreting CIMT measurements are the effects of age, sex, and ethnicity. In general, the CIMT increases in a linear fashion approximately 0.008 mm/y in the general population between the ages of 45 and 85 years.[70] However, CIMT increases more per year in patients with increased serum cholesterol levels and clinically evident atherosclerosis.[71] In addition, men typically have increased CIMT in comparison with women.[71,72] For instance, the mean CIMT value for African American women 65 years of age is reported to be 0.75 mm, whereas for African American men the mean value is 0.86 mm.[68] The carotid intima medial layer is reportedly thicker in African Americans than in white or Asian people. Smoking, increased systolic blood pressure, and increased LDL levels are also associated with increased CIMT.[71] However, despite these well-known variations of CIMT measurement in different populations, many studies report cutoff points that were chosen a priori for simplicity.[5]

Although CIMT is strongly associated with atherosclerosis, increased CIMT is not a specific finding for atherosclerosis. Other inflammatory disorders such rheumatoid arthritis or Takayasu arteritis may cause thickening of the carotid intima media layers.[73]

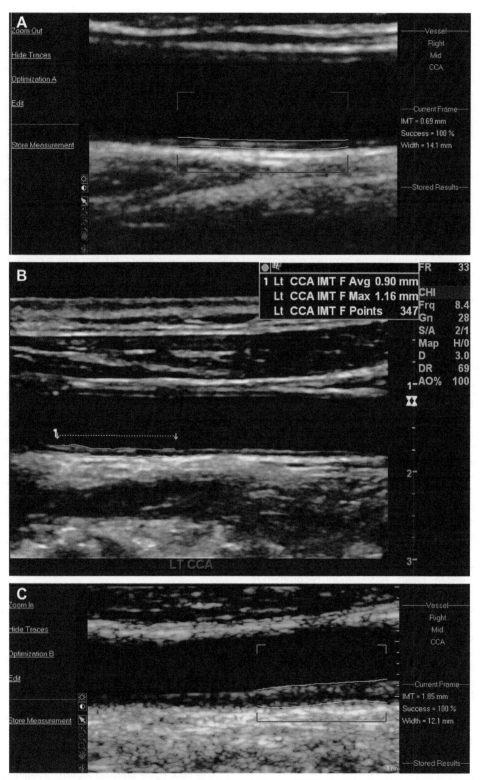

Fig. 7. Semiautomated measurement of the carotid intima thickness. (*A*) Semiautomated measurement of the mid–right common carotid artery for 1.4 cm. The CIMT is normal at 0.69 mm. (*B*) In this patient, the CIMT is slightly thickened, measuring 0.9 cm, with a maximum measurement of 1.16 mm. (*C*) This patient has a markedly increased CIMT, measuring 1.85 mm for 1.21 cm in the mid–right common carotid artery. (*A* and *C Courtesy of* Philips Healthcare; with permission.)

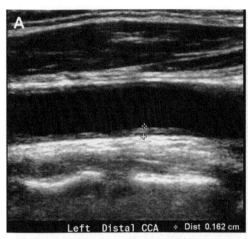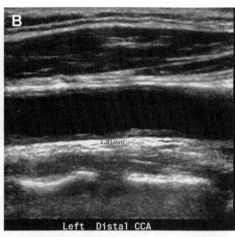

Fig. 8. Interobserver and intraobserver variability. Hand-placed calipers. (*A*) Sagittal gray-scale image of the left common carotid artery showing incorrect placement of calipers for measuring CIMT. Not only is the crosshair of the more anterior caliper misplaced above the echogenic intima-luminal interface but it is not directly over the lower caliper, thus giving an elongated tangential measure. (*B*) Repeat measurement of the CIMT from the left common carotid artery in the same patient as in (*A*) shows that the CIMT measures 1.01 mm rather than 1.62 mm.

CURRENT RECOMMENDATIONS REGARDING MEASUREMENT OF CIMT

In 2000, the Prevention Conference V of the American Heart Association concluded that, in asymptomatic persons more than 45 years old, carefully performed carotid ultrasound examination with CIMT measurement can add incremental information to traditional risk factor assessment.[49] In 2006, the Screening for Heart Attack Prevention and Education Task Force recommended treatment strategies, such as more aggressive LDL reduction, based on risk stratification in patients with very high risk (CIMT≥1 mm or 75th percentile) versus patients with moderately high risk (CIMT<1 mm or 50–75th percentile).[74] Currently, the American Heart Association recommends that CIMT be measured as part of the clinical risk assessment for atherosclerosis.[47] Several publications have discussed approaches to modify risk classification as traditionally calculated using models like the Framingham Risk Score based on CIMT measurement.[60,66,69,75] However, these approaches have never been validated in longitudinal cohort studies. In addition, one of the fundamental criticisms of the use of CIMT measurement as a marker for CVD risk is that, although it is an excellent epidemiologic tool, application to individual patients in clinical practice outside the research setting is difficult because of a lack of standardized protocols and reporting criteria. Nevertheless, progress is being made in this regard and consensus statements on standards for acquisition, measurement, and reporting CIMT data have been published or are pending.[66,76,77]

In 2008, the American Society of Echocardiography (ASE) Carotid Intima-Media Thickness Task Force published consensus guidelines derived from 4 large epidemiologic studies that reported CIMT values in percentiles by age, sex, and race.[66] The ASE task force consensus statement suggests that measuring CIMT and identifying carotid plaque is useful for refining CVD risk assessment in patients with intermediate CVD risk, that is, in patients with a 6% to 20% 10-year risk of MI or death from CAD, but without documented CAD or coronary disease risk equivalent conditions.[66] Specifically, the ASE task force identified the following clinical circumstances in which CIMT measurement was most likely to be useful[1]: individuals with a family history of premature CVD in a first-degree relative[2]; individuals less than 60 years old with severe abnormality of a single risk factor who otherwise would not be candidates for pharmacotherapy; or[3] women less than 60 years old with at least 2 CVD risk factors.[66] The task force considered that the presence of carotid plaque or CIMT greater than or equal to the 75th percentile for the patient's age, sex, and race indicates increased CVD risk and is a possible indication of the need for more aggressive risk-reduction interventions.[66]

The task force advised against imaging for the sole purpose of assessing CVD risk in patients with established atherosclerotic vascular disease or if the results would not be expected to alter therapy.[66] In addition, serial CIMT measurements to address progression or regression of athero-sclerosis were not recommended for use in clinical practice at this time,[66] although some investiga-tors do suggest performing annual evaluations if abnormal results are found, and every 2 to 5 years if results are normal.[68]

According to ASE guidelines, CIMT measure-ment should be performed as part of a thorough scan of the extracranial carotid arteries for the presence of carotid plaques to achieve maximum sensitivity for identifying subclinical vascular disease.[66] The carotid arteries should be evalu-ated using a linear-array transducer operating at a fundamental frequency of at least 7 MHz with B-mode imaging and state-of-the-art equipment using standard protocols (see American Institute of Ultrasound in Medicine [AIUM], ACR, or In-tersocietal Commission for the Accreditation of vascular Laboratories [ICVAL] guidelines). On high-resolution gray-scale imaging, the wall of the CCA shows 3 distinct layers (see Fig. 1). Cen-trally, an echogenic linear layer representing the intima and the interface of the intima with the arte-rial lumen is observed. Underneath this, a hypoe-choic layer is believed to represent the media. Beneath the media, there is another echogenic linear layer representing the adventitia and inter-face with the surrounding soft tissues. In total, this gives the appearance of 2 parallel echogenic lines separated by a more hypoechoic area. Although atherosclerosis and CIMT progress more rapidly in the bulb and ICA segments, CIMT measurement should be made from the far wall of the distal 1 cm of the CCA. The vessel should be straight and horizontal on the image (ie, perpendicular to the insonating US beam).

Patients should be scanned at a standard depth of 4 cm if possible. The typical pixel size when imaging at a 4-cm depth is approximately 0.11 mm. Because CIMT measurements are extremely small, differences of 1 digital pixel can classify patients in different risk categories, so close atten-tion to instrumentation, standardized imaging, measurement technique (see Fig. 8), and reading protocols is critical. Because carotid wall thick-ening is not uniform, a single value as measured with hand-held calipers (see Fig. 6) may not accu-rately represent arterial changes. Hence, multiple measurements of several extended segment lengths of at least 1 cm with leading-edge-to-leading-edge methodology (see Fig. 7) not only gives a better overall assessment of the CIMT but is also more reproducible with less interob-server and intraobserver variability.[66] Most of the previously described studies used a manual technique to measure CIMT, but the ASE task force specifically recommended the use of a vali-dated semiautomated border-detection computer program that allows manual adjustments of the tracked borders to improve reproducibility and shorten examination time (Fig. 9), although the investigators acknowledge that computer-based programs generally measure CIMT slightly larger than manual measurement, including manually performed leading edge measurements. Seg-ments should be measured in triplicate and from 3 angles (lateral, anterior, and posterior; all differing by 45°). Any value differing by more than 0.05 mm should be excluded. CIMT values are then averaged and mean CIMT values reported. Some laboratories recommend measuring CIMT in multiple segments and reporting a maximum

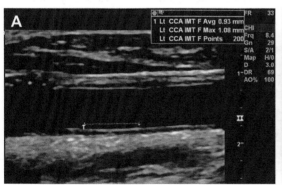
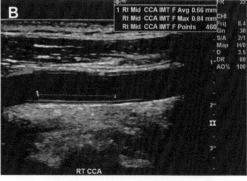

Fig. 9. Manual adjustment of border edge-detection computer programming. Although most investigators consider that automated measurement of the CIMT for a 1-cm length of the common carotid artery reduces both interobserver and intraobserver variability, computer-generated measurement of the CIMT remains an imper-fect standard and, in most cases, generates a slightly larger measurement of CIMT than is obtained with caliper measurements. In addition, manual override capability is recommended to enhance accuracy. For example, the line corresponding to the adventitia-media interface is extremely irregular in (A). Repeat measurement with manual override in (B) allows straightening of the posterior line, allowing more accurate measurement of the CIMT.

value or the mean of maximum values (**Fig. 10**) as well, although this was not specifically recommended in the ASE guidelines. The CIMT from the posterior walls of the right and left CCA are reported separately. Any focal area of plaque in a segment of the CCA being measured should be included in the measurement. In addition, specific training should be required for all sonographers measuring CIMT.

Despite the perception that accurate measurement of CIMT is easy, most investigators report considerable intraobserver and interobserver variability. Some of the most common pitfalls and approaches to minimizing them are described later. Measurements should not be made if the echogenic interface between the intima and the lumen is not clearly seen (**Fig. 11**). To improve visibility, adjusting the focal zone, increasing the gain, and ensuring that the vessel is truly horizontal to the transducer are the most helpful techniques to improve resolution. In addition, the CIMT should only be measured if the double echogenic lines representing the intima-media interface and advential interface can be seen in the near wall as well as the posterior wall, even though the near wall is not routinely measured; his will ensure that the center of the vessel is being scanned and a true CIMT measurement is obtained that is not exaggerated by inclusion of the curvature of the lateral wall. If it is only possible to clearly see a segment of CIMT for less than 1 cm, a shorter segment can be measured. If the CCA is too deep (>4 cm), gentle compression of the overlying soft tissues or a different angle of interrogation can be attempted. If the vessel is too shallow (<4 cm), image degradation caused by slice thickness artifact or near-field artifact may occur and a standoff pad or thick application of gel can be tried. If the

vessel is tortuous, extending the neck or turning to the contralateral side may be helpful to straighten the CCA. Using the zoom feature is not recommended, and the use of intravenous ultrasound contrast is not recommended for clinical assessment of CIMT at this time.

The ASE task force recommended communicating CIMT results by qualitatively describing broad ranges of percentiles.[66] CIMT values greater than or equal to the 75th percentile are considered high and indicate increased CVD risk. Values in the 25th to 75th percentiles are considered average and indicate unchanged CVD risk. Values less than or equal to the 25th percentile are considered lower CVD risk, but whether or not they justify less-aggressive preventive therapy than standard care is not known.[66]

The United States Centers for Medicare and Medicaid has established a Current Procedural Terminology code (0126T) for "Common CIMT study for evaluation of atherosclerotic burden or coronary heart disease risk factor assessment."[66] Texas is currently the only state with legislation that mandates health insurance reimbursement for CIMT, whereas hospitals and clinics charge patients between $160 and $325 for interpretation.[68]

THE FUTURE TRENDS

Much research is currently focused on the identification of vulnerable plaque, that is, hemorrhagic and/or inflammatory plaque that is more likely to rupture and thereby expose thrombogenic material within the central core of the plaque to the blood stream, precipitating thromboembolic events resulting in MI and/or stroke. Recently published histologic studies have clearly shown that

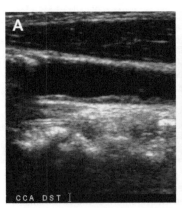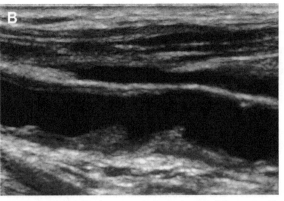

Fig. 10. (*A, B*) Irregularity of the carotid intima media layer. Sagittal gray-scale images of 2 different patients with extremely irregular thickening of the carotid intima media layers. Whether it is more accurate or has more clinical significance to report the mean measurement for a 1-cm length of the vessel wall versus the maximum thickness, which would be different in these 2 patients, is not known. Reporting methodology is variable in most large trials.

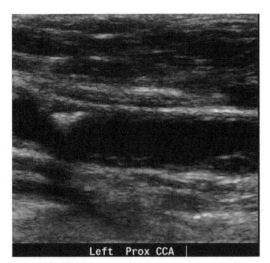

Fig. 11. Incomplete visualization of the carotid intima media layer. In this patient, although the CIMT looks thickened, the echogenic linear interface between the intima and the vessel lumen is not continuously visible. Therefore, this image is not adequate for CIMT measurement.

an increase in plaque neovascularity as well as increased density of the advential vasa vasorum are established features of vulnerable plaque.[78–80] Several investigators have convincingly shown that increased contrast enhancement of plaque in the ICAs on late-phase intravenous contrast-enhanced US correlates with increased plaque neovascularity, and thus may serve as a surrogate marker for vulnerable plaque.[29,81,82] In addition, in 2006, Feinstein[29] speculated that a decrease in contrast enhancement in carotid plaque on late-phase intravenous contrast-enhanced US could be documented in patients responding to statin therapy. More recently, several investigators have reported that patients with symptomatic carotid plaque show increased intraplaque contrast enhancement in comparison with asymptomatic plaque on late-phase intravenous contrast-enhanced US.[83–85] These investigators also showed that the increased contrast enhancement in plaque occurred in areas of plaque that were hypoechoic on gray-scale imaging, confirming prior reports that hypoechoic plaque is more likely to be hemorrhagic or vulnerable (discussed earlier). Furthermore, Staub and colleagues[85] found that contrast enhancement of plaque on US was also directly associated with the severity of carotid artery stenosis. Although these series involved only a small number of patients, it is possible that late-phase contrast enhancement of carotid plaque on US may become a useful screen for vulnerable plaque and will be useful in

risk stratification of patients with hypoechoic or extensive plaque. Perhaps contrast enhancement of plaque will prove helpful in determining which patients with greater than or equal to 70% ICA stenosis or ICA stenoses in the 50% to 69% range are at most risk for stroke and, therefore, will benefit from intervention.

Elastography is also being evaluated as a means of identifying vulnerable plaque. Lipid-laden plaque and hemorrhagic plaque might be expected to be more compressible than calcified, stable plaque, although less compressible than the normal arterial wall. Plaque that is compressible might also be expected to show more radial strain. Decreased elasticity of plaque might expose the plaque to increased inward strain and higher stress, predisposing the plaque to rupture.[86] However, the data have been conflicting to date[86,87] and the clinical usefulness of plaque elastograms, which provide information regarding radial strain and shear distribution, is yet to be determined.

Arterial stiffness can also be assessed in various ways with US,[88] including pulse wave velocity[89]; change in diameter during the cardiac cycle; distensibility, compliance, and circumferential stress of the vessel wall[86]; pulsatility index[90]; and brachial artery reactivity testing.[65] Arterial stiffness has been shown to be correlated with hypertension, diabetes, and CVD events[65,86,88–90] However, most of these techniques remain research tools at the present time and the optimal, most reliable method of measuring arterial stiffness is not known.

SUMMARY

A growing body of evidence has validated sonographic evaluation of CIMT as a surrogate marker for atherosclerosis and risk of cardiovascular event. In addition, measurement of CIMT has been shown in the research setting to be useful in assessing disease progression, and may also be used as an effective, easily measurable end point in clinical trials evaluating therapeutic efficacy of medications and lifestyle changes, such as weight loss and exercise, intended to reduce CVD risk. However, although CIMT has been proved to be an independent risk factor for CVD, whether or not the clinical usefulness of CIMT measurement substantially exceeds that of traditional CVD risk models such as the Framingham Risk Score or the SCORE model has not been fully proven because outcome analysis studies have yet to be performed to determine whether improved risk prediction obtained from CIMT measurements and carotid plaque imaging translates into improved CVD outcomes.[13,66] Hence, the clinical practice recommendations put forth by the ASE are based solely on observational data. Controversies remain regarding methodology of measurement and reporting. Although multiple large multicenter trials have reported consistent association of increased CIMT with cardiovascular disease risk, the method of measuring and reporting CIMT differed in most of these trials and both intraobserver and interobserver variability exists no matter what protocol is used when measuring a structure that is so small and close in size to the limit of the spatial resolution of even state-of-the-art ultrasound equipment. In the absence of consistency, most clinical centers favor the methodology proposed by the ASE.[66] However, new consensus guidelines describing methodology and reporting, as well as who should be screened, are expected to be proposed by the Society of Atherosclerosis Imaging and Prevention in the near future.

REFERENCES

1. Thom T, Haase N, Rosamond W, et al, American Heart Association Statistics Committee and Stroke Statistics Subcommittee. Heart disease and stroke statistics–2006 update: a report from the American Heart Association Statistics Committee and Stroke Statistics Subcommittee. Circulation 2006;113:e85–151 [erratum in: Circulation 2006;11;113:e696. Circulation 2006;114:e630].

2. WHO Factsheet No. 317. Updated September 2009. Available at: http://who.int/mediacentre/factsheets/fs317/en. Accessed September 18, 2010.

3. Azen SP, Mack WJ, Cashin-Hemphill L, et al. Progression of coronary artery disease predicts clinical coronary events. Long-term follow-up from the Cholesterol Lowering Atherosclerosis Study. Circulation 1996;93:34–41.

4. McGill HC Jr, McMahan CA, Malcom GT, et al. Effects of serum lipoproteins and smoking on atherosclerosis in young men and women. The PDAY Research Group. Pathobiological Determinants of Atherosclerosis in Youth. Arterioscler Thromb Vasc Biol 1997; 17:95–106.

5. Chambless LE, Heiss G, Folsom AR, et al. Association of coronary heart disease incidence with carotid arterial wall thickness and major risk factors: the Atherosclerosis Risk in Communities (ARIC) Study, 1987-1993. Am J Epidemiol 1997;146:483–94.

6. Khot UN, Khot MB, Bajzer CT, et al. Prevalence of conventional risk factors in patients with coronary heart disease. JAMA 2003;290:898–904.

7. Hodis HN, Mack WJ, LaBree L, et al. The role of carotid arterial intima-media thickness in predicting clinical coronary events. Ann Intern Med 1998;128:262–9.

8. Kastelein JJ, de Groot E. Ultrasound imaging techniques for the evaluation of cardiovascular therapies. Eur Heart J 2008;7:849–58.

9. Cao JJ, Arnold AM, Manolio TA, et al. Association of carotid artery intima-media thickness, plaques, and C-reactive protein with future cardiovascular disease and all-cause mortality: the Cardiovascular Health Study. Circulation 2007;116:32–8.

10. Salonen JT, Salonen R. Ultrasonographically assessed carotid morphology and the risk of coronary heart disease. Arterioscler Thromb 1991;11:1245–9.

11. O'Leary DH, Polak JF, Kronmal RA, et al. Carotid-artery intima and media thickness as a risk factor for myocardial infarction and stroke in older adults. Cardiovascular Health Study Collaborative Research Group. N Engl J Med 1999;340:14–22.

12. Lorenz MW, Markus HS, Bots ML, et al. Prediction of clinical cardiovascular events with carotid intima-media thickness: a systematic review and meta-analysis. Circulation 2007;115:459–67.

13. Lorenz MW, Schaefer C, Steinmetz H, et al. Is carotid intima media thickness useful for individual prediction of cardiovascular risk? Ten-year results from the Carotid Atherosclerosis Progression Study (CAPS). Eur Heart J 2010;31:2041–8.

14. Stein JH, Fraizer MC, Aeschlimann SE, et al. Vascular age: integrating carotid intima-media thickness measurements with global coronary risk assessment. Clin Cardiol 2004;27:388–92.

15. Davignon J, Ganz P. Role of endothelial dysfunction in atherosclerosis. Circulation 2004;109:III27.

16. Brevetti G, Martone VD, de Cristofaro T, et al. High levels of adhesion molecules are associated with impaired endothelium-dependent vasodilation in patients with peripheral arterial disease. Thromb Haemost 2001;85:63.

17. Massberg S, Brand K, Gruner S, et al. A critical role of platelet adhesion in the initiation of atherosclerotic lesion formation. J Exp Med 2002;196:887–96.

18. Cybulsky MI, Gimbrone MA Jr. Endothelial expression of a mononuclear leukocyte adhesion molecule during atherogenesis. Science 1991;251:788–91.

19. Leitinger N. Oxidized phospholipids as modulators of inflammation in atherosclerosis. Curr Opin Lipidol 2003;14:421–30.

20. Skalen K, Gustafsson M, Rydberg EK, et al. Subendothelial retention of atherogenic lipoproteins in early atherosclerosis. Nature 2002;417:750–4.

21. Smith JD, Trogan E, Ginsberg M, et al. Decreased atherosclerosis in mice deficient in both macrophage colony-stimulating factor (op) and apolipoprotein E. Proc Natl Acad Sci U S A 1995;92:8264–8.

22. Peiser L, Mukhopadhyay S, Gordon S. Scavenger receptors in innate immunity. Curr Opin Immunol 2002;14:123–8.

23. Janeway CA Jr, Medzhitov R. Innate immune recognition. Annu Rev Immunol 2002;20:197–216.

24. Hansson GK. Inflammation, atherosclerosis and the coronary artery. N Engl J Med 2005;352:1685–95.

25. Bjorkbacka H, Kunjathoor VV, Moore KJ, et al. Reduced atherosclerosis in MyD88-null mice links elevated serum cholesterol levels to activation of innate immunity signaling pathways. Nat Med 2004; 10:416–21.

26. Perschinka H, Mayr M, Millonig G, et al. Cross-reactive B-cell epitopes of microbial and human heat shock protein 60/65 in atherosclerosis. Arterioscler Thromb Vasc Biol 2003;23:1060–5.

27. Streblow DN, Soderberg-Naucler C, Viera J, et al. The human cytomegalovirus chemokine receptor US28 mediates vascular smooth muscle cell migration. Cell 1999;99:511–20.

28. Soderberg-Naucler C, Emery VC. Viral infections and their impact on chronic renal allograft dysfunction. Transplantation 2001;71(Suppl 11):SS24–30.

29. Feinstein SB. Contrast ultrasound imaging of the carotid artery vasa vasorum and atherosclerotic plaque neovascularization. J Am Coll Cardiol 2006;48: 236–43.

30. Ross R. Atherosclerosis – an inflammatory disease. N Engl J Med 1999;340:115–26.

31. Saba L, Sanfilippo R, Montisci R, et al. Associations between carotid artery wall thickness and cardiovascular risk factors using multidetector CT. AJNR Am J Neuroradiol 2010;31:1758–63.

32. Stary HC, Chandler AB, Dinsmore RE, et al. A definition of advanced types of atherosclerotic lesions and a histological classification of atherosclerosis: a report from the committee on Vascular Lesions of the Council on Arteriosclerosis, American Heart Association. Circulation 1995;92:1355–74.

33. Jonasson L, Holm J, Skalli O, et al. Regional accumulations of T cells, macrophages and smooth muscle cells in the human atherosclerotic plaque. Arteriosclerosis 1986;6:131–8.

34. Kovanen PT, Kaartinen M, Paavonen T. Infiltrates of activated mast cells at the site of coronary atheromatous erosion or rupture in myocardial infarction. Circulation 1995;92:1084–8.

35. Schoenhagen P, Ziada KM, Kapadia SR, et al. Extent and direction of arterial remodeling in stable versus unstable coronary syndromes: an intravascular ultrasound study. Circulation 2000;101:598–603.

36. Davies MJ. Stability and instability: two faces of coronary atherosclerosis: the Paul Dudley White lecture 1995. Circulation 1996;94:2013–20.

37. Falk E, Shah PK, Fuster V. Coronary plaque disruption. Circulation 1995;92:657–71.

38. Glagov S, Weisenberg E, Zarins CK, et al. Compensatory enlargement of human atherosclerotic coronary arteries. N Engl J Med 1987;316:1371–5.

39. Bluth EI, Kay D, Merritt CR, et al. Sonographic characterization of carotid plaque: detection of hemorrhage. AJR Am J Roentgenol 1986;146:1061–5.

40. Reilly LM, Lusby RJ, Hughes L, et al. Carotid plaque histology using real-time ultrasonography. Clinical and therapeutic implications. Am J Surg 1983;146: 188–93.

41. O'Donnell TF, Erodes L, Mackey WC, et al. Correlation of B-mode ultrasound imaging and arteriography with pathologic findings at carotid endarterectomy. Arch Surg 1985;120:443–5.

42. Sterpetti AV, Schultz RD, Feldhaus RJ, et al. Ultrasonographic features of carotid plaque and the risk of subsequent neurologic deficits. Surgery 1988;104: 652–60.

43. Leahy AL, McCollum PT, Feeley TM, et al. Duplex ultrasonography and selection of patients for carotid endarterectomy: plaque morphology or luminal narrowing? J Vasc Surg 1988;8:558–62.

44. Polak JF, Shemanski L, O'Leary DH, et al. Hypoechoic plaque at US of the carotid artery: an independent risk factor for incident stroke in adults aged 65 years or older. Radiology 1998;208:649–54.

45. Topol EJ, Nissen SE. Our preoccupation with coronary luminology. The dissociation between clinical and angiographic findings in ischemic heart disease. Circulation 1995;92:2333–42.

46. Sankatsing RR, de Groot E, Jukema JW, et al. Surrogate markers for atherosclerotic disease. Curr Opin Lipidol 2005;16:434–41.

47. Smith SC, Greenland P, Grundy SM. Prevention Conference V: Beyond secondary prevention: identifying the high-risk patient for primary prevention. Circulation 2000;101:111–6.

48. O'Leary DH, Polak JF. Intima-media thickness: a tool for atherosclerosis imaging and event prediction. Am J Cardiol 2002;90:18–21.

49. Greenland P, Abrams J, Aurigemma GP, et al. Prevention Conference V: Beyond secondary prevention: identifying the high-risk patient for primary prevention: noninvasive tests of atherosclerotic burden: Writing Group III. Circulation 2000;101:E16–22.

50. Bots ML, Grobbee DE. Intima media thickness as a surrogate marker for generalised atherosclerosis. Cardiovasc Drugs Ther 2002;16:341–51.

51. Polak JF, Funk LC, O'Leary D. Inter-reader difference in common carotid artery intima media thickness. J Ultrasound Med 2011;30:915–20.

52. Pignoli P, Tremoli E, Poli A, et al. Intimal plus medial thickness of the arterial wall: a direct measurement with ultrasound imaging. Circulation 1986;74:1339–406.

53. Bots ML, Hoes AW, Koudstaal PJ, et al. Common carotid intima-media thickness and risk of stroke and myocardial infarction: the Rotterdam Study. Circulation 1997;96:1432–7.

54. Bots ML, Baldassarre D, Simon A, et al. Carotid intima-media thickness and coronary atherosclerosis: weak or strong relations? Eur Heart J 2007; 28:398–406.

55. Mattace-Raso F, van Popele NM, Schalekamp MA, et al. Intima-media thickness of the common carotid arteries is related to coronary atherosclerosis and left ventricular hypertrophy in older adults. Angiology 2002;53:569–74.

56. Taylor AJ, Sullenberger LE, Lee HJ, et al. Arterial Biology for the Investigation of the Treatment Effects of Reducing Cholesterol (ARBITER) 2: a double-blind, placebo-controlled study of extended-release niacin on atherosclerosis progression in secondary prevention patients treated with statins [erratum in: Circulation 2005;111:e446. Circulation 2004;110:3615]. Circulation 2004;110:3512–7 [Epub 2004 Nov 10].

57. Crouse JR, Raichlen JS, Riley WA, et al, METEOR Study Group. Effect of rosuvastatin on progression of carotid intima-media thickness in low-risk individuals with subclinical atherosclerosis: the METEOR Trial. JAMA 2007;297:1344–53.

58. Lester SJ, Eleid MF, Khandheria BK, et al. Carotid intima-media thickness and coronary artery calcium score as indications of subclinical atherosclerosis. Mayo Clin Proc 2009;84:229–33.

59. Eleid MF, Lester SJ, Wiedenbeck TL, et al. Carotid ultrasound identifies high risk subclinical atherosclerosis in adults with low Framingham Risk Scores. J Am Soc Echocardiogr 2010;23:802–8.

60. Junyent M, Zambón D, Gilabert R, et al. Carotid atherosclerosis and vascular age in the assessment of coronary heart disease risk beyond the Framingham Risk Score. Atherosclerosis 2008;196:803–9.

61. Polak JF, Pencia MJ, Pencina KM, et al. Carotid-wall intima-media thickness and cardiovascular events. N Engl J Med 2011;365:213–21.

62. Taylor AJ, Kent SM, Flaherty PJ, et al. Arterial Biology for the Investigation of the Treatment Effects of Reducing Cholesterol: a randomized trial comparing the effects of atorvastatin and prevastatin on carotid intima medial thickness. Circulation 2002; 106(16):2055–60.

63. Espeland MA, O'Leary DH, Terry JG, et al. Carotid intimal-media thickness as a surrogate for cardiovascular disease events in trials of HMG-CoA reductase inhibitors. Curr Control Trials Cardiovasc Med 2005;6:3.

64. Wong M, Edelstein J, Wollman J, et al. Ultrasonic-pathological comparison of the human arterial wall. Verification of intima-media thickness. Arterioscler Thromb 1993;13:482–6.

65. Roman MJ, Naqvi TZ, Gardin JM, et al. Clinical application of noninvasive vascular ultrasound in cardiovascular risk stratification: a report from the American Society of Echocardiography and the Society of Vascular Medicine and Biology. J Am Soc Echocardiogr 2006;19(8):943–54.

66. Stein JH, Korcarz CE, Hurst RT, et al, American Society of Echocardiography Carotid Intima-Media Thickness Task Force. Use of carotid ultrasound to identify subclinical vascular disease and evaluate cardiovascular disease risk: a consensus statement from the American Society of Echocardiography Carotid Intima-Media Thickness Task Force. Endorsed by the Society for Vascular Medicine [erratum in: J Am Soc Echocardiogr 2008;21:376]. J Am Soc Echocardiogr 2008;21:93–111.

67. O'Leary DH, Polak JF, Kronmal RA, et al. Distribution and correlates of sonographically detected carotid artery disease in the Cardiovascular Health Study. The CHS Collaborative Research Group. Stroke 1992;23:1752–60.

68. Cobble M, Bale B. Carotid intima-media thickness: knowledge and application to everyday practice. Postgrad Med 2010;122:10–8.

69. Gepner AD, Wyman RA, Korcarz CE, et al. An abbreviated carotid intima-media thickness scanning protocol to facilitate clinical screening for subclinical atherosclerosis. J Am Soc Echocardiogr 2007;20:1269–75.

70. Howard G, Burke GL, Szko M, et al. Does the association of risk factors and atherosclerosis change with age? An analysis of the combined ARIC and CHS cohorts. The Atherosclerosis Risk in Communities (ARIC) and Cardiovascular Health Study (CHS) investigators. Stroke 1997;28:1693–701.

71. Polak JF. Carotid intima-media thickness. Ultrasound Q 2009;25:55–61.

72. Poli A, Tremoli E, Colombo A, et al. Ultrasonographic measurement of the common carotid artery wall thickness in hypercholesterolemic patients. A new model for the quantization and follow-up of preclinical atherosclerosis in living human subjects. Atherosclerosis 1988;70:253–61.

73. Rodriguez R, Gómez-Díaz RA, Tanus Haj J, et al. Carotid intima-media thickness in pediatric type 1 diabetic patients. Diabetes Care 2007;30:2599–602.

74. Naghavi M, Falk E, Hecht HS, et al, SHAPE Task Force. From vulnerable plaque to vulnerable patient–Part III: executive summary of the Screening for Heart Attack Prevention and Education (SHAPE) Task Force report. Am J Cardiol 2006;98:2H–15H.

75. Bard RL, Kalsi H, Rubenfire M, et al. Effect of carotid atherosclerosis screening on risk stratification during primary cardiovascular disease prevention. Am J Cardiol 2004;93:1030–2.

76. Mintz GS, Nissen SE, Anderson WD, et al. American College of Cardiology Clinical Expert Consensus Document on Standards for Acquisition, Measurement and Reporting of Intravascular Ultrasound Studies (IVUS). A report of the American College of Cardiology Task Force on Clinical Expert Consensus Documents. J Am Coll Cardiol 2001;37: 1478–92.

77. Touboul PJ, Hennerici MG, Meairs S, et al. Mannheim carotid intima-media thickness consensus

(2004-2006). An update on behalf of the Advisory Board of the 3rd and 4th Watching the Risk Symposium, 13th and 15th European Stroke Conferences, Mannheim, Germany, 2004, and Brussels, Belgium, 2006. Cerebrovasc Dis 2007;23:75–80.

78. McCarthy MJ, Loftus IM, Thompson MM, et al. Angiogenesis and the atherosclerotic carotid plaque: an association between symptomatology and plaque morphology. J Vasc Surg 1999;30(2):261–8.

79. Dunmore BJ, McCarthy MJ, Naylor AR, et al. Carotid plaque instability and ischemic symptoms are linked to immaturity of microvessels within plaques. J Vasc Surg 2007;45(1):155–9.

80. Moreno PR, Purushothaman KR, Fuster V, et al. Plaque neovascularization is increased in ruptured atherosclerotic lesions of human aorta: implications for plaque vulnerability. Circulation 2004;110(14):2032–8.

81. Coli S, Magnoni M, Sangiorgi G, et al. Contrast enhanced ultrasound imaging of intraplaque neovascularization in carotid arteries: correlation with histology and plaque echogenicity. J Am Coll Cardiol 2008;52(3):223–30.

82. Neems RF, Goldin M, Dainauskas J, et al. Real-time contrast enhanced ultrasound imaging of the neovascularization within the human carotid plaque. J Am Coll Cardiol 2004;43:374A.

83. Xiong L, Deng YB, Zhu Y, et al. Correlation of carotid plaque neovascularization detected by using contrast-enhance US with clinical symptoms. Radiology 2009;251:583–9.

84. Owen DR, Shalhoulb J, Miller S, et al. Inflammation within carotid atherosclerotic plaque: assessment with late-phase contrast enhanced US. Radiology 2010;255:638–44.

85. Staub D, Partovi S, Schinkel AF, et al. Correlation of carotid atherosclerotic lesion echogenicity and severity at standard US with intraplaque neovascularization detected at contrast-enhanced US. Radiology 2011;258:618–26.

86. Beaussier H, Masson I, Collin C. Carotid plaque, arterial stiffness gradient, and remodeling in hypertension. Hypertension 2008;52:729–36.

87. Schmitt C, Soulez G, Maurice RL, et al. Noninvasive vascular elastography: toward a complementary characterization tool of atherosclerosis in carotid arteries. Ultrasound Med Biol 2007;33:1841–58.

88. Laurent S, Cockcroft J, Bortel LV, et al. Expert consensus document on arterial stiffness: methodological issues and clinical applications. Eur Heart J 2006;27:2588–605.

89. Laurent S, Boutouyrie P. Arterial stiffness: a new surrogate end point for cardiovascular. J Nephrol 2007;20:S45–50.

90. Fukuhara T, Hida K. Pulsatility index at the cervical internal carotid artery as a parameter of microangiopathy in patients with type 2 diabetes. J Ultrasound Med 2006;25:599–605.

Pitfalls in Carotid Ultrasound Diagnosis

Beverly E. Hashimoto, MD

KEYWORDS

- Carotid stenosis • Carotid ultrasound • Carotid arteries
- Internal carotid artery • Ultrasound

Every year, about 800,000 people develop either a new or recurrent stroke and about 135,000 die of the disease.[1] About 20% of strokes are attributed to extracranial carotid artery stenosis.[2] Carotid ultrasound has long been established as a useful screening study for evaluation of extracranial carotid disease. Three meta-analyses reviewing published data concluded that the sensitivity range of the technique is 86% to 94% and the specificity range is 87% to 94%.[2–4]

Although these published carotid ultrasound results are high, the accuracy in general laboratories may be lower. A meta-analysis reviewing both published and private data found lower results: sensitivity 83%, specificity 54%.[5] Investigators attributed the lower accuracy rates to less publication bias and introduction of data that reflect everyday clinical practice. To obtain data, the investigators advertised in professional societies and made private inquiries to professional colleagues. Only about one-third of the patients in this meta-analysis were found in published trials. The rest of the data resulted from unpublished audits from individuals or organizations in which carotid sonography was directly compared either with angiography or with another noninvasive study such as computed tomography (CT) or magnetic resonance (MR) angiography. This lower accuracy rate in routine practice suggests that performance and interpretation of carotid ultrasound is not always straightforward. Unavoidable variability between ultrasound and other modalities has been shown to be caused by differences between physiologic (Doppler) data and anatomic (contrast angiography, MR angiography, CT angiography) information.[6–9] In recognition of this variability, standardized protocols include linking a range of anatomic stenoses with a range of internal carotid artery (ICA) spectral values. Doppler criteria of ICA stenosis have been published by an interdisciplinary consensus conference.[10,11]

However, despite extensive dissemination of carotid sonographic performance criteria and interpretation,[10–12] performance of the examination varies.[13] Even imagers with extensive experience produce errors.[14] Radiologists and sonographers who perform vascular examinations are commonly familiar with grayscale and color Doppler technique, but less familiar with pulse wave Doppler performance. Because a significant part of the carotid Doppler interpretation is based on the spectral waveform, consistent production of an accurate waveform is critical to the examination. This article focuses on some of the most common reasons for misinterpretation of the carotid spectral waveform.

TECHNICAL PITFALLS

Technical pitfalls result either from suboptimal operator technique or from difficulties with the patient or the patient's anatomy. Potential technical problems include (1) poorly trained technologists, (2) unreliable equipment, (3) inappropriate frequency or transducer, (4) inappropriate sonographic gain, (5) large sample volume, (6) large Doppler angle, (7) heavily calcified arteries, (8) tortuous artery, and (9) external carotid artery (ECA) mistaken for ICA.

Similar to other sonographic techniques, carotid ultrasound is highly operator dependent. A crucial method to avoid interpretive errors is to retain only

Disclosure: Dr Beverly Hashimoto is an equipment consultant for GE Medical Systems.
Noninvasive Vascular Laboratory, Department of Radiology, Virginia Mason Medical Center, C5-XR, 1100 9th Avenue, Seattle, WA 98111, USA
E-mail address: Beverly.hashimoto@vmmc.org

1556-858X/11/$ – see front matter © 2011 Elsevier Inc. All rights reserved.

highly trained vascular technologists. Inadequate examination of the carotid system by poorly trained technologists may lead to serious errors in interpretation.[14] This inadequate evaluation usually results from either lack of meticulous evaluation of the arteries or poor sonographic technique resulting in suboptimal visualization of sections of the vessels. To avoid missing a stenosis, the sonographer should routinely scan the arteries in a systematic manner such as starting inferiorly in the proximal common carotid artery (CCA), and proceeding superiorly to the distal ICA. The sonographer should not skip sections of the vessel. Furthermore, the sonographer should extend the examination as far distally as possible.

Even if the operator is skilled, poor equipment produces poor spectral results. Multiple studies have reported that equipment from different vendors produce slightly different results.[13,15,16] Although vascular laboratories are generally careful about acquiring and maintaining equipment, validation of equipment results is commonly not performed regularly. Without periodic validation, poor equipment will not be identified. The Asymptomatic Carotid Atherosclerosis Study (ACAS) validation study found that about 20% of 63 devices from 27 ACAS centers showed no statistical relationship between Doppler velocity and percent stenosis.[17] This study further implied that dependence on the reputation of a vendor was not directly related to good vascular equipment performance. Of 4 manufacturers that had at least 8 devices in the study, each manufacturer had at least 1 machine with excellent sensitivity and 1 with poor sensitivity.[17] Therefore, as part of quality control of carotid ultrasound, the radiologist should identify consistent performance of all vascular equipment. Besides determining discrepancies between carotid ultrasound examinations and

other modalities, the radiologist should also keep a record of which equipment is associated with each discrepancy. If one machine is disproportionately involved in these discrepancies, then the radiologist can focus more attention on the machine's performance by side-by-side testing with other machines or by contacting the vendor for evaluation. In general, if the laboratory has modern equipment, there should not be any significant differences in equipment accuracy.

Carotid ultrasound is performed with a linear transducer with intermediate Doppler frequencies (such as 8–4 MHz),[18] whereas the grayscale imaging of the carotid arteries may require higher frequencies because the carotid arteries are superficially located in the neck. Doppler shift signals are weaker, so intermediate frequencies usually provide optimal signal strength for producing a spectral waveform. If extremely low (<3 MHz) frequencies or small aperture transducers are used, the Doppler signal may be distorted and produce inaccurate velocity measurements (**Fig. 1**).

When documenting the spectral waveform, the vascular technologist should be trained in correctly adjusting the pulse Doppler gain. If the gain is too low, the waveform will be too faint and difficult to measure. If the gain is too high, there will be increased noise in the spectral image and the radiologist may misinterpret the pattern as increased spectral broadening or turbulence. If the physician notes severe spectral broadening and the grayscale and color Doppler images do not show the reason for the turbulence, then the radiologist should review the pulse wave Doppler gain setting, which is usually on the image (**Fig. 2**).

When performing the carotid ultrasound examination, the sonographer should use a small Doppler sample volume; generally the smallest volume available on the machine. In a normal

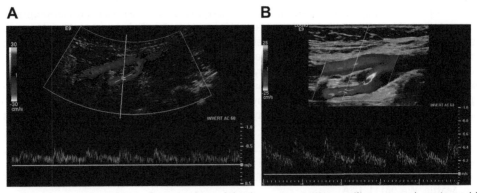

Fig. 1. Duplex Doppler examination of a normal ICA. (*A*) When a 1 to 5 MHz curvilinear transducer is used for the duplex carotid examination, the waveform is distorted. (*B*) Duplex carotid examination illustrates the ICA waveform of the same patient as in (*A*) with an appropriate transducer (6–9 MHz linear).

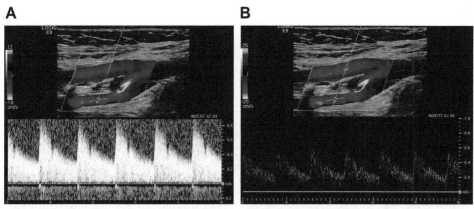

Fig. 2. Duplex Doppler examination of a normal ICA. (*A*) When the pulse Doppler gain is inappropriately increased, there is increased artifact throughout the spectral waveform. (*B*) Duplex ICA waveform of the same patient as in (*A*) with an appropriate gain setting.

vessel, a small sample volume produces a thin spectral waveform. If the sample volume is inadvertently increased, this increase in sample volume allows documentation of a wider range of red cell velocities so the waveform thickens and there may appear to be spectral broadening (**Fig. 3**).[18,19]

Applying a low Doppler angle is important in obtaining accurate results. The importance of the Doppler angle is shown by the Doppler equation:

$$F = AV\cos\theta$$

where F is the Doppler frequency shift; A is a constant; V is the velocity of red blood cells (RBC); θ is the angle between RBC and the Doppler beam angle. As the Doppler angle approaches 90°, the Doppler signal decreases to zero. Therefore, large Doppler angles produce inaccurate, low spectral waveforms (**Fig. 4**). For best results, the Doppler angle should be less than or equal to 60°.[10,11] However, to best quantify an irregular stenosis or a tortuous vessel, smaller angles are applied as necessary. Doppler angle is always documented on the images, allowing for comparison if a discrepancy is identified on follow-up examination. Researchers examining the impact on velocity measurements produced by variations in angle noted that, as long as transducer settings such as sample volume size, wall filter, and Doppler gain are kept constant between measurements, then small changes in angle are not significant.[20]

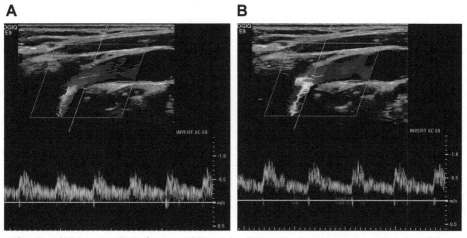

Fig. 3. Duplex Doppler examination of a normal ICA. (*A*) A large sample volume results in a waveform with spectral broadening simulating turbulence. (*B*) Duplex waveform of the same patient as in (*A*) with small sample volume.

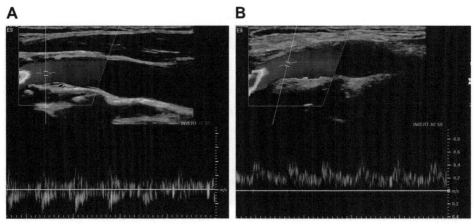

Fig. 4. Duplex Doppler examination of a normal ICA. (*A*) When the pulse Doppler angle is 88°, the Doppler signal is low. (*B*) Duplex ICA waveform of the same patient as in (*A*) with 60° angle.

Heavily calcified arteries may compromise Doppler interrogation. Usually, the operator can adjust the angle of the transducer to adequately evaluate the artery, but severe calcification may obscure arterial flow (**Fig. 5**). Investigators have suggested that, when the plaque calcification obscures a high-grade lesion for more than 1 cm, the velocity beyond the calcification may not reflect the severity of the stenosis.[21] Whenever heavy calcification significantly interferes with the examination, this limitation should be documented and the radiologist should indicate this issue in the interpretation, so additional imaging may be necessary to completely evaluate the carotid lumen.[10,11]

Tortuous arteries may exhibit turbulent flow with increased velocities. If the interpreter only reviews the velocity data, the imager may misinterpret an otherwise normal tortuous vessel as a stenotic one. Color-flow Doppler is a valuable method to clarify the cause of abnormally increased velocities when no significant luminal stenosis can be identified (**Fig. 6**).[14,22]

Occasionally, the ECA may be mistaken for the ICA. Diagnostically, this error is serious when one of these vessels is severely stenotic or occluded. Inexperienced imagers may incur this error when identification of these vessels is solely based on anatomic location. Although the ECA is usually medial and anterior to the ICA, vascular radiologists should identify these vessels by their waveform patterns, not their location.[23] Characteristics that distinguish the ECA from the ICA include (1) the ECA has branches, (2) ECA systolic waveform has a larger slope (sharper upstroke), (3) ECA has a narrower systolic peak, (4) ECA has lower diastolic flow, and (5) temporal tap of the superficial temporal artery superimposes a wavy pattern on the ECA waveform.[24] When initially faced with distinguishing the ECA from the ICA, technologists can use color Doppler to identify small branches from the ECA.[22] However, in experienced laboratories, mistaking the ECA for the ICA generally only occurs if these arteries have extremely abnormal flow patterns. The greatest challenge in distinguishing between the ECA and the ICA is when the ECA exhibits high diastolic flow, sometimes termed internalization of the ECA. If this pattern is present, there is usually severe stenosis or occlusion of the ICA, so the ECA is providing collateral flow. In this situation, the temporal tap is a useful method to clarify the identity of the ECA (**Fig. 7**).[25–27]

SPECTRAL WAVEFORM PITFALLS

Several clinical and physiologic circumstances produce arterial waveforms that lead to misinterpretation. These situations include (1) stenosis outside the sonographic field of view, (2) tight stenosis with trickle flow, (3) high-flow or low-flow states, (4) overcall stenosis on side contralateral to true stenosis or occlusion, and (5) postinterventional states. When the stenosis is outside the sonographic field of view, the carotid ultrasound may be unaffected: the waveforms are unremarkable. A known pitfall of carotid ultrasound is inability to identify intracranial stenoses.[28] However, when the occlusion or severe stenosis is either proximal or distal to the region of insonation, waveforms in the adjacent carotid artery sometimes exhibit significant abnormalities. By understanding these characteristic waveform changes, radiologists can identify significant stenosis either proximal or distal to the site of the examination. When the

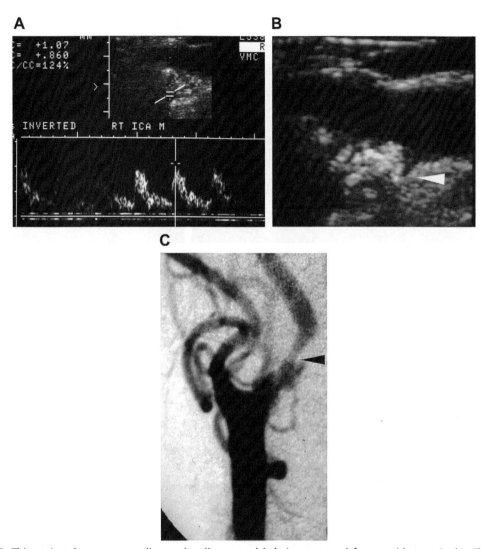

Fig. 5. This patient has severe cardiovascular disease and is being screened for carotid stenosis. (*A, B*): Pulse Doppler shows less than a 50% stenosis (ICA peak systolic velocity [PSV] is 107 cm/s/s, ICA/CCA ratio is 1.2) but the ICA is heavily calcified and only a short section is visible (*arrowhead*). (*C*) Because the examination was limited, angiography was performed, which revealed a 68% stenosis by NASCET (North American Symptomatic Carotid Endarterectomy Trial) criteria (*arrowhead*).[56,57] Calcification obscured this stenosis for the carotid ultrasound examination.

stenosis is proximal to the site of insonation, the carotid waveform exhibits a low systolic velocity and a delayed, blunted systolic peak velocity (**Fig. 8**).[29,30] If the stenosis is distal, then the carotid waveform shows a large systolic slope (sharp upstroke), and low or no diastolic flow (**Fig. 9**). If a distal carotid occlusion is suspected, the radiologist should evaluate the study to identify whether the flow in the CCA goes to zero at end diastole and whether there is a thump or a short waveform with a low systolic velocity and no diastolic flow. These findings are commonly associated with occlusion.[18]

Near occlusion may be difficult to differentiate sonographically from occlusion. Although sonography is highly accurate for occlusion, carotid sonography is less sensitive for near occlusion. Studies have found that, although carotid ultrasound detects about 100% of occlusions, sonography identifies between 85% and 95% of near occlusions.[30–34] Erroneously interpreting a near occlusion as an occlusion is potentially a serious error because patient therapy differs between these conditions. If extremely low-velocity flow or velocities that are not equivalent to the severity of stenosis depicted by color or power Doppler

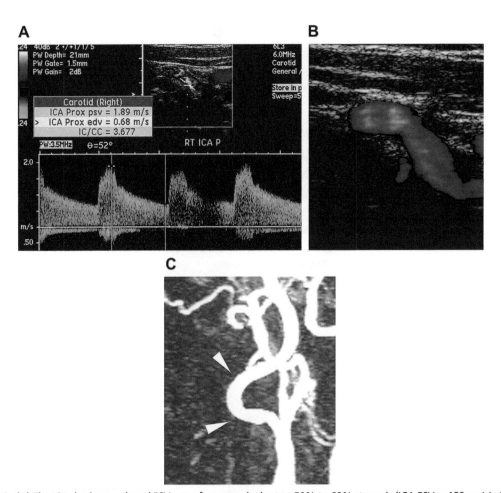

Fig. 6. (*A*) The ICA duplex produced PSV waveforms equivalent to 50% to 69% stenosis (ICA PSV = 189 cm/s/s; ICA/CCA = 3.7). (*B*) However, the color Doppler examination showed severe tortuosity without evidence of significant stenosis. (*C*) Angiography confirmed severe tortuosity (*arrowheads*) without significant stenosis (stenosis = 25% by NASCET).

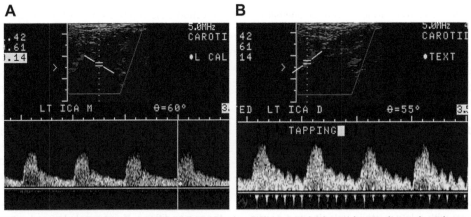

Fig. 7. (*A*) During this carotid examination, only 1 vessel was discovered. The wide systolic peak and presence of diastolic flow suggested that the vessel was the ICA. (*B*) However, temporal tap clearly identified the vessel as the ECA. The ICA was occluded.

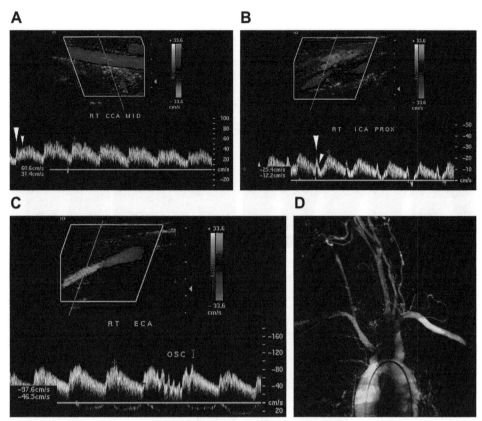

Fig. 8. A 57-year-old man presents with right-sided amaurosis fugax and innominate artery disease. (*A*) Spectral waveforms from right CCA show flat, blunted appearance. Systolic spikes (*large arrowhead*) and midsystolic deceleration (*small arrowhead*) are subtleties present in several cardiac cycles. (*B*) Spectral waveforms from right ICA show findings typical present with innominate artery stenosis. These abnormalities include sharp systolic spikes (*large arrowhead*) and marked midsystolic deceleration (*small arrowhead*) with flow to baseline during several cardiac cycles. PROX, proximal. (*C*) Spectral waveforms from right ECA show high diastolic flow with a resistive index of 0.52. Temporal tap producing transient oscillations (OSC) identify this vessel as the ECA. Unlike the CCA and ICA, the ECA waveforms do not clearly show systolic spike or midsystolic deceleration. (*D*) Antero-posterior view from conventional digital subtraction angiogram shows focal eccentric high-grade innominate artery stenosis. (*Courtesy of* Dr Edward Grant and the American Roentgen Ray Society; with permission; and *From* Grant EG, El Saden S, Madrazo B, et al. Innominate artery occlusive disease: sonographic findings. AJR Am J Roentgenol 2006;186(2):394–400; with permission.)

imaging are identified, then a near-occlusive lesion should be considered. Color or power Doppler is also useful to identify a flow channel (**Fig. 10**).[21,22,28,31,33,35] If no Doppler signal is identified in the carotid, occlusion may be present. The previously described Doppler thump associated with careful pulse and color Doppler insonation of the vessel strongly indicate occlusion. However, lack of Doppler signal may also be caused by suboptimal technique or insensitive equipment.[36] If no Doppler flow is identified, then additional imaging is recommended to either confirm occlusion or identify near occlusion. Although the gold standard for near occlusion is angiography,[37]

researchers have found that contrast-enhanced MR angiography is an excellent alternative method to identify near occlusion.[38,39]

Interpretation of carotid ultrasound in patients who experience either high or low cardiovascular flow states is difficult. The carotid velocities are strongly biased by the underlying abnormal blood flow condition. In high-flow states, the nonstenotic velocity of the carotids is much higher than normal. The interpreter needs to rely more on the change of velocity within the ICA if a stenosis is suspected. If the ICA stenotic velocity is twice the prestenotic ICA velocity, then at least a 50% stenosis should be suspected. An ICA/CCA ratio greater than 4

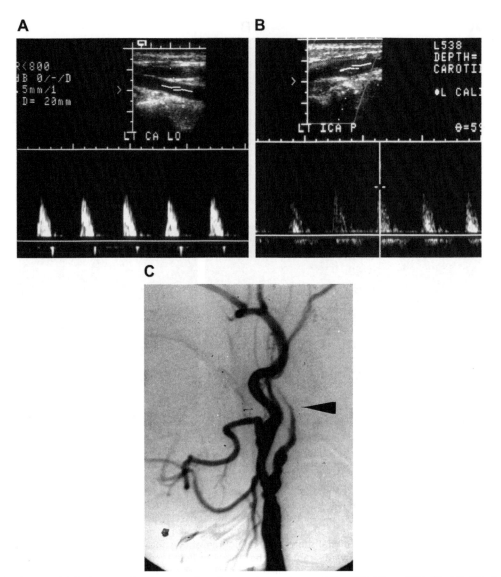

Fig. 9. The carotid duplex examination revealed abnormal waveforms of the CCA (*A*) and ICA (*B*). (*A*) CCA shows absence of diastolic flow. (*B*) ICA reversal of flow in diastole and sharp systolic upstroke of ICA waveform suggested distal stenosis. (*C*) CT angiography showed an occlusion of ICA (*arrowhead*).

should suggest a greater than 70% stenosis. Additional information including a narrow lumen by color Doppler and grayscale imaging and the presence of a poststenotic waveform with spectral broadening should guide the radiologist.[10,11]

Low-flow states are more difficult than high-flow states because the extremely low velocities may be difficult to measure.[10,11] Although stenoses should increase the carotid velocities, the increase may be difficult to detect.[24] Color Doppler signal in these patients may be poor because of the low-velocity flow and gray scale may not be useful if the thrombus is acute and appears anechoic

or severely hypoechoic or calcified. If the study appears limited, then additional imaging is appropriate (**Fig. 11**).

Overcalling stenosis in the carotid artery contralateral to a severely stenotic or occluded carotid is one of the most common carotid ultrasound diagnostic errors.[14] When one carotid is occluded or severely stenotic, the contralateral carotid artery peak systolic velocity (PSV) commonly increases.[40–42] This PSV increase has been called compensatory flow. Investigators have suggested that this increase of velocity is caused by collateral flow from the normal ICA to the contralateral side.

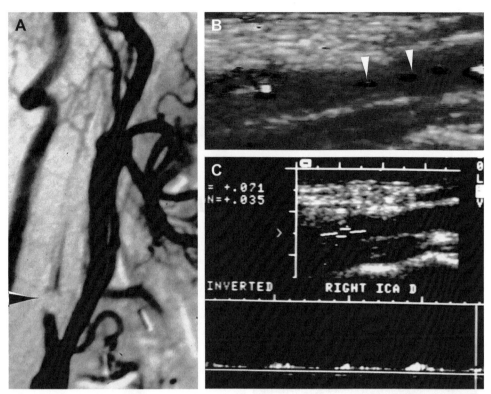

Fig. 10. Initial pulse Doppler carotid ultrasound did not identify flow within the ICA. Color Doppler was not used. (*A*) Conventional arteriogram showed severe stenosis (*arrowhead*). After arteriogram was performed, the patient was reexamined sonographically. (*B*) Color Doppler showed trickle flow within the ICA (*arrowheads*). (*C*) Duplex Doppler confirmed the low flow associated with the tight stenosis. In this case, color Doppler would have been useful to initially identify the tight stenosis.

However, published reports provide conflicting evidence for this hypothesis.[43]

In the presence of compensatory ICA flow, the increased velocity may be complicated by turbulence from mild plaque. If the radiologist only evaluates the ICA waveform, then the imager may erroneously interpret these findings as a significant stenosis. This pitfall can be avoided if the radiologist examines the pattern of PSV increase, ICA/CCA ratio, and color Doppler and grayscale lumen images of the high-velocity segment. Unlike focal stenosis, compensatory flow is associated with velocity increase throughout a vessel. Furthermore, if the ICA/CCA ratio is not increased by more than 2 and the anatomic images are not consistent with the PSV, then the radiologist should conclude that the increased PSV is caused by compensatory flow (**Fig. 12**).

To avoid interpretation errors, the radiologist should be aware of the usual vascular changes that develop after carotid interventional procedures such as carotid endarterectomy (CEA) or

carotid angioplasty and stent placement (CAS) (**Fig. 13**). After CEA, about 10% to 15% of post-CEA carotid arteries have restenosis (>50%) by spectral velocity criteria. Two-thirds never become clinically significant; most of these so-called stenoses regress.[44–46] In CEA vessels that show regression, the apparent stenosis probably represented normal postoperative vascular change. Shortly after CEA, the lack of intimalization results in higher turbulence (spectral broadening). If there is tortuosity, this turbulence may be associated with increased PSVs and simulate a stenosis. If increased velocities are present in a carotid that has been treated with endarterectomy, color Doppler is a useful method to clarify whether the spectral information is accurate. Restenosis after CAS has been found to be 4% after 1 year and 6% after 2 years for studies using restenosis threshold of 50% to 70%, and 6% after 1 year and 7.5% after 2 years for those using a threshold of 70% to 80%.[47] After CAS, multiple investigators have found that there is increased carotid PSV in

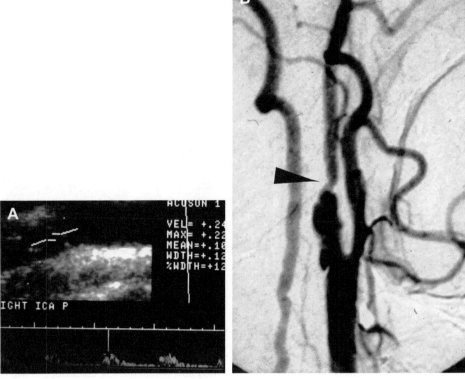

Fig. 11. (*A*) Duplex Doppler of patient with extremely low cardiac output showed very low peak systolic velocities (<30 cm/s/s) throughout the ICA. (*B*) Because the patient's low-flow state limited the carotid ultrasound, angiogram was performed, which showed a significant ICA stenosis (*arrowhead*).

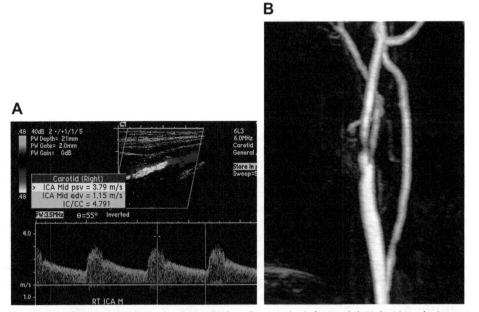

Fig. 12. Duplex Doppler and MR angiogram identified no flow in the left ICA. (*A*) Right ICA velocity parameters were consistent with greater than 70% stenosis (ICA PSV = 378 cm/s/s, ICA/CCA ratio = 4.8). However, the increased velocity is not focal but is evident throughout the ICA, as illustrated by the presence of aliasing throughout the vessel. (*B*) MR angiogram showed that right ICA had only 50% stenosis by NASCET. This case showed compensatory ICA flow in the left ICA, causing abnormal increase of velocities.

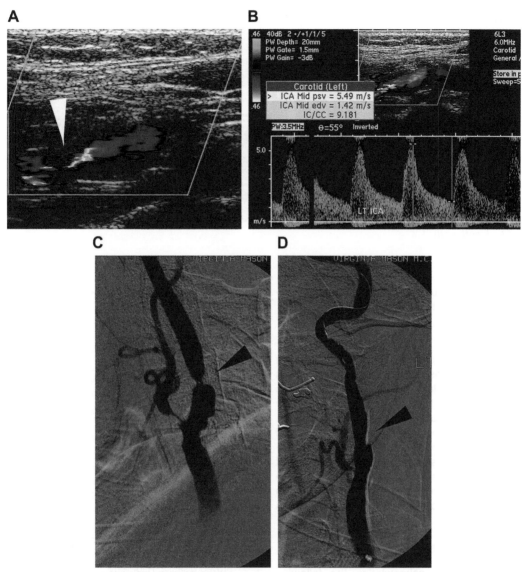

Fig. 13. Carotid ultrasound of a 78-year-old man with recent right-sided weakness. (*A*) Color Doppler and (*B*) duplex ultrasound show a greater than 70% stenosis. (*C*) Angiogram confirmed severe stenosis (*arrowhead*) and (*D*) CAS was subsequently performed. (*E*) After CAS, color Doppler and (*F*) duplex ultrasound show no significant stenosis.

the nonstenotic stented segment.[48–55] The velocity increase in intrastent stenosis has been attributed to increased wall stiffness.[51,55]

In conjunction with increased velocities in nonstenotic stented vessels, researchers have also confirmed that ICA velocity and ICA/CCA ratio for intrastent stenosis are higher than comparable nonstented carotid stenosis. Investigators report that ICA velocities greater than 175 to 240 cm/s/s and ICA/CCA ratios greater than 2.5 to 3.8

correspond with intrastent stenoses between 50% and 70%. Furthermore, ICA velocities greater than 300 to 450 cm/s/s and ICA/CCA ratios greater than 3.8 to 4.75 correspond with intrastent stenoses greater than or equal to 70% stenosis.[48–54] Although various investigators have reported stent-specific velocity and ratio thresholds for their own laboratories, there is no current clinical consensus defining a specific protocol. Until a consensus is reached, each laboratory should

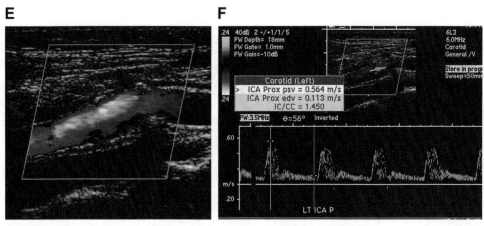

Fig. 13. (*continued*)

monitor its carotid ultrasound stent data and internally validate a protocol.

SUMMARY

Most errors in interpreting carotid ultrasound may be avoided if the vascular laboratory carefully hires well-trained vascular technologists, monitors its technical skills, and buys and maintains high-quality sonographic vascular equipment. Furthermore, the radiologist should be familiar with ICA and ECA waveforms and understand how to differentiate between these vessels when they exhibit abnormal flow patterns. Color Doppler is an important method to avoid mistakes that result from normal physiologic increase of ICA and CCA velocities.

ACKNOWLEDGMENTS

I would like to acknowledge the following personnel: Morris Ferensen for processing my images; Suzy Murray-Dirks, Lindsay Oram, and Stacy Buck for assisting in providing clinical imaging; and Erin Turpin for editorial assistance.

REFERENCES

1. Lloyd-Jones D, Adams RJ, Brown TM, et al. Heart disease and stroke 2010 update: a report from the American Heart Association. Circulation 2010;121: e46–215.
2. Wolff T, Guirguis-Blake J, Miller T, et al. Screening for carotid artery stenosis: an update of the evidence for the U.S. Preventive Services Task Force. Ann Intern Med 2007;147:860–70.
3. Jahromi AS, Cina CS, Liu Y, et al. Sensitivity and specificity of color duplex ultrasound measurement in the estimation of internal carotid artery stenosis: a systematic review and meta-analysis. J Vasc Surg 2005;41:962–72.
4. Nederkoorn PJ, van der Graaf Y, Hunink M. Duplex ultrasound and magnetic resonance angiography compared with digital subtraction angiography in carotid artery stenosis. Stroke 2003;34:1324–32.
5. Cappell FM, Wardlaw JM, Young GR, et al. Carotid artery stenosis: accuracy of noninvasive tests—individual patient data meta-analysis. Radiology 2009; 251:493–502.
6. Grant EG, Duerinckx AJ, El Saden SM, et al. Ability to use duplex US to quantify internal carotid arterial stenoses: fact or fiction? Radiology 2000;214:247–52.
7. Vergara M. Duplex US for the estimation if internal carotid stenosis [letter]. Radiology 2001;219:575–6.
8. Lee VS, Hertzberg BS, Workman MJ, et al. Variability of Doppler us measurements along the common carotid artery: effects on estimates of internal carotid arterial stenosis in patients with angiographically proved disease. Radiology 2000;214:387–92.
9. Shaalan WE, Wahlgren CM, Desai T, et al. Reappraisal of velocity criteria for carotid bulb/internal carotid artery stenosis utilizing high-resolution B-mode ultrasound validated with computed tomography angiography. J Vasc Surg 2008;48:104–13.
10. Grant EG, Benson CB, Moneta GL, et al. Carotid artery stenosis: grayscale and Doppler ultrasound diagnosis—society of radiologists in ultrasound consensus conference. Ultrasound Q 2003;19:190–8.
11. Grant EG, Benson CB, Moneta GL, et al. Carotid artery stenosis: gray-scale and Doppler US diagnosis—society of radiologists in ultrasound consensus conference. Radiology 2003;229:340–6.
12. Jaff MR, Goldmakher GV, Lev MH, et al. Imaging of the carotid arteries: the role of duplex ultrasonography, magnetic resonance arteriography, and computerized tomographic arteriography. Vasc Med 2008;13: 281–91.

13. Crittenden JJ. Extreme variability of cerebrovascular US results and some solutions [letter]. Radiology 1997;205:577–9.

14. Horrow MM, Stassi J, Shurman A, et al. The limitations of carotid sonography: interpretive and technology-related errors. AJR Am J Roentgenol 2000;174:189–94.

15. Fillinger MF, Baker RJ, Zwolak RM, et al. Carotid duplex criteria for a 60% or greater angiographic stenosis: variation according to equipment. J Vasc Surg 1996;24:856–64.

16. Kuntz KM, Polak JF, Whittemore AD, et al. Duplex ultrasound criteria for the identification of carotid stenosis should be laboratory specific. Stroke 1997;28:597–602.

17. Howard G, Baker WH, Chambless LE, et al. An approach for the use of Doppler ultrasound as a screening tool for hemodynamically significant stenosis (despite heterogeneity of Doppler performance). Stroke 1996;27:1951–7.

18. Standness DE. Extracranial arterial disease. In: Duplex scanning in vascular disorders. New York: Raven Press; 1990. p. 92–120.

19. Van Merode T, Hick P, Hoeks AP, et al. Limitations of Doppler spectral broadening in the early detection of carotid artery disease due to the size of the sample volume. Ultrasound Med Biol 1983;9:581–6.

20. Thomas N, Taylor P, Padayachee S. The impact of theoretical errors on velocity estimation and accuracy of duplex grading of carotid stenosis. Ultrasound Med Biol 2003;28:191–6.

21. Erickson SJ, Mewissen MW, Foley WD, et al. Stenosis of the internal carotid artery: assessment using color Doppler imaging compared with angiography. AJR Am J Roentgenol 1989;152:1299–305.

22. Hallam MJ, Reid JM, Cooperberg PL. Color-flow Doppler and conventional duplex scanning of the carotid bifurcation: prospective double-blind, correlative study. AJR Am J Roentgenol 1989;152:1101–5.

23. Diethrich EB. Normal cerebrovascular anatomy and collateral pathways. In: Zwiebel WJ, Pellerito JS, editors. Introduction to vascular ultrasonography. 5th edition. New York: Elsevier Saunders; 2005. p. 133–42.

24. Zwiebel WJ. Normal findings and technical aspects of carotid sonography. In: Zwiebel WJ, Pellerito JS, editors. Introduction to vascular ultrasonography. 5th edition. New York: Elsevier Saunders; 2005. p. 143–54.

25. Zwiebel WJ, Pellerito JS. Carotid occlusion, unusual carotid pathology, and tricky carotid cases. In: Zwiebel WJ, Pellerito JS, editors. Introduction to vascular ultrasonography. 5th edition. New York: Elsevier Saunders; 2005. p. 173–89.

26. Budorick NE, Rojratanakiat W, O'Boyle MK, et al. Digital tapping of the superficial temporal artery: significance in carotid duplex sonography. J Ultrasound Med 1996;15:459–64.

27. Klierwer MA, Freed KS, Hertzberg BS, et al. Temporal artery tap: usefulness and limitations in carotid sonography. Radiology 1996;201:481–4.

28. Eliasziw M, Rankin RN, Fox AJ, et al. Accuracy and prognostic consequences of ultrasonography in identifying severe carotid artery stenosis. Stroke 1995;26:1747–52.

29. Mitchell EL, Moneta GL. Ultrasound assessment of carotid stenosis. In: Zwiebel WJ, Pellerito JS, editors. Introduction to vascular ultrasonography. 5th edition. New York: Elsevier Saunders; 2005. p. 173–89.

30. Schmidt P, Sliwka U, Simon SG, et al. High-grade stenosis of the internal carotid artery assessed by color and power Doppler imaging. J Clin Ultrasound 1998;26:85–9.

31. Berman SS, Devine JJ, Erdoes LS, et al. Distinguishing carotid artery pseudo-occlusion with color-flow Doppler. Stroke 1995;26(3):434–8.

32. Furst G, Saleh A, Wenserski F, et al. Reliability and validity of noninvasive imaging of internal carotid artery pseudo-occlusion. Stroke 1999;30:1444–9.

33. Mansour MA, Mattos MA, Hood DB, et al. Detection of total occlusion, string sign, and preocclusive stenosis of the internal carotid artery by color-flow duplex scanning. Am J Surg 1995;170:154–8.

34. Bowman JN, Olin JW, Teodorescu VJ, et al. Carotid artery pseudo-occlusion: does end-diastolic velocity suggest need for treatment? Vasc Endovascular Surg 2009;43:374–8.

35. Sidhu PS, Allan PL. Ultrasound assessment of internal carotid artery stenosis [Review II]. Clin Radiol 1997;52:654–8.

36. Romero JM, Lev MH, Chan ST, et al. US of neurovascular occlusive disease: interpretive pearls and pitfalls. Radiographics 2002;22:1165–76.

37. Fox AJ, Eliasziw M, Rothwell PM, et al. Barnett HJM for the North American Symptomatic Carotid Endarterectomy Trial and European Carotid Surgery Trial Groups. Identification, prognosis, and management of patients with carotid artery near occlusion. AJNR Am J Neuroradiol 2005;26:2086–94.

38. Hammond CJ, McPherson SJ, Patel JV, et al. Assessment of apparent internal carotid occlusion on ultrasound: prospective comparison of contrast-enhanced ultrasound, magnetic resonance angiography and digital subtraction angiography. Eur J Vasc Endovasc Surg 2008;35:405–12.

39. El-Saden SM, Grant EG, Hathout GM, et al. Imaging of the internal carotid artery: the dilemma of total versus near total occlusion. Radiology 2001;221:301–8.

40. Henderson RD, Steinman DA, Eliasziw M, et al. Effect of contralateral carotid artery stenosis on carotid ultrasound velocity measurements. Stroke 2000;31:2636–40.

41. AbuRahma AF, Richmond BK, Robinson PA, et al. Effect of contralateral severe stenosis or carotid

occlusion on duplex criteria of ipsilateral stenosis: comparative study of various duplex parameters. J Vasc Surg 1995;22:751–62.

42. Heijenbrok-Kal MH, Nederkoorn PJ, Buskens E, et al. Diagnostic performance of duplex ultrasound in patients suspected of carotid artery disease: the ipsilateral versus contralateral artery. Stroke 2005; 36:2105–9.

43. Beckett WW, Davis PC, Hoffman JC. Duplex Doppler sonography of the carotid artery: false-positive results in an artery contralateral to an artery with marked stenosis. AJNR Am J Neuroradiol 1990;11: 1049–53.

44. Samson RH, Showalter DP, Yunis JP, et al. Hemodynamically significant early recurrent carotid stenosis: an often self-limiting and self-reversing condition. J Vasc Surg 1999;30:446–52.

45. Golledge J, Cuming R, Ellis M, et al. Duplex imaging findings predict stenosis after carotid endarterectomy. J Vasc Surg 1997;26:43–8.

46. Skelly CL, Meyerson SL, Curi MA, et al. Routine early postoperative duplex scanning is unnecessary following uncomplicated carotid endarterectomy. Vasc Endovascular Surg 2002;36:115–22.

47. Groschel K, Riecker A, Schulz JB, et al. Systematic review of early recurrent stenosis after carotid angioplasty and stenting. Stroke 2005;36:367–73.

48. AbuRahma AF, Abu-Halimah S, Bensenhaver J, et al. Optimal carotid duplex velocity criteria for defining the severity of carotid in-stent restenosis. J Vasc Surg 2008;48:589–94.

49. Chi YW, White CJ, Woods TC, et al. Ultrasound velocity criteria for carotid in-stent restenosis. Catheter Cardiovasc Interv 2007;69:349–54.

50. Lal BK, Hobson RW, Tofighi B, et al. Duplex ultrasound velocity criteria for the stented carotid artery. J Vasc Surg 2008;47:63–73.

51. Lal BK, Hobson RW, Goldstein J, et al. Carotid artery stenting: is there a need to revise ultrasound velocity criteria? J Vasc Surg 2004;39:58–66.

52. Setacci C, Chisci E, Setacci F, et al. Grading carotid intrastent restenosis. Stroke 2008;39:1189–96.

53. Stanziale SF, Wholey MH, Boules TN, et al. Determining in-stent stenosis of carotid arteries by duplex ultrasound criteria. J Endovasc Ther 2005; 12:346–53.

54. Zhou W, Felkai DD, Evans M, et al. Ultrasound criteria for severe in-stent restenosis following carotid artery stenting. J Vasc Surg 2008;47:74–80.

55. Nederkoorn PJ, Brown MM. Optimal cut-off criteria for duplex ultrasound for the diagnosis of restenosis in stented carotid arteries: review and protocol for a diagnostic study. BMC Neurol 2009;9:36.

56. North American Symptomatic Carotid Endarterectomy Trial: methods, patient characteristics, and progress. Stroke 1991;22:711–20.

57. Fox AJ. How to measure carotid stenosis. Radiology 1993;186:316–8.

Dialysis Grafts and Fistulae: Planning and Assessment

Heidi R. Umphrey, MD*, Mark E. Lockhart, MD, MPH,
Carl A. Abts, RDMS, Michelle L. Robbin, MD

KEYWORDS

- Ultrasound • Hemodialysis access • Arteriovenous fistula
- Arteriovenous graft • Preoperative ultrasound mapping

During 2009, approximately 573,000 patients were being treated for end-stage renal disease in the United States[1]; approximately 355,000 patients received hemodialysis in 2008.[1] Vascular access procedures and associated complications are a major cause of morbidity and increasing health care cost in patients undergoing hemodialysis.[2] There are 2 types of permanent hemodialysis access: the autogenous arteriovenous fistula (AVF) and the synthetic arteriovenous graft (graft). Mature AVFs (suitable for hemodialysis) are associated with a decreased frequency of thrombosis and infection when compared with grafts, and therefore are preferred for hemodialysis.[3–5] Several institutions have shown that preoperative sonographic evaluation can alter surgical planning and increase the successful creation of AVFs.[6–9] Ultrasonography may be able to serve as a surrogate for AVF maturation.[10,11] Studies disagree whether close access monitoring with early detection and intervention improves access longevity.[12–23] Evaluation of the problem AVF and graft, assessing for stenosis or other treatable causes of AVF nonmaturation and graft dysfunction, has been described.[24,25] This review describes our institution's sonographic approaches for hemodialysis access planning and subsequent access assessment.

ULTRASONOGRAPHIC TECHNIQUE

Our sonographic evaluation of hemodialysis access planning and assessment has been previously reported, but technical details to optimize the evaluation are expanded here.[11,26,27] Most of the examination should be performed with the patient sitting upright with their arm comfortably resting on a towel on a procedure stand or phlebotomy table. The arm is positioned approximately 45° from the body (**Fig. 1**). This positioning allows for adequate filling and distention of the veins within the arm. The supine position is used for optimal evaluation of the internal jugular and subclavian veins, again to optimally fill the veins.

Gray Scale

The highest-frequency transducer that adequately penetrates the tissue should be used, because near-field gray-scale resolution increases with increased frequency. Generally a linear array transducer 12 to15 MHz or higher is preferred. A small footprint probe such as a hockey-stick style can be useful for ease of evaluation. If increased penetration is needed, it is preferable to decrease the frequency of the initial high-frequency probe before switching to a lower-frequency probe. Patients with increased soft tissue or deeper vessels such as the brachial artery or subclavian veins may need a lower-frequency transducer (5–12 MHz) for good resolution at a greater depth. Advanced imaging features such as harmonic and compound imaging may also improve vascular wall detail for a given frequency.

If a central venous stenosis is suspected because of absent or decreased transmitted cardiac pulsatility or respiratory phasicity, a small

Department of Radiology, University of Alabama at Birmingham, 619 19th Street South, Birmingham, AL 35294-6830, USA
* Corresponding author.
E-mail address: humphrey@uabmc.edu

1556-858X/11/$ – see front matter © 2011 Elsevier Inc. All rights reserved.

ultrasound.theclinics.com

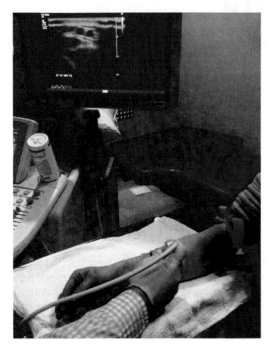

Fig. 1. Optimal patient positioning for upper extremity ultrasonography to access for hemodialysis access.

footprint probe in the 5-MHz to 8-MHz range may be used to improve visualization of the brachiocephalic vein or superior vena cava in the parasternal region or suprasternal notch. The focal zone should be adjusted so that gray-scale resolution is optimized for the vessel of interest (**Fig. 2**) and the image depth should be reduced so that the vessel fills much of the image space. Minimal transducer pressure should be applied to the skin so as not to deform the vessel of interest (**Fig. 3**).

Color and Spectral Doppler

For optimal color Doppler assessment, a presumed normal region of vessel should be evaluated. The color gain should be increased until pixels of color are seen outside the wall of the vessel, and subsequently the gain is decreased until color is seen only within the vessel lumen (**Fig. 4**). The velocity scale should be adjusted until color fills the entire lumen of the vessel without color bleeding (pixels of color displayed outside the vessel lumen) (see **Fig. 4**). The color scale should be adjusted such that aliasing does not occur. Color Doppler aliasing is seen when color in the vessel wraps around the scale from highest to lowest color (**Fig. 5**). Vessels without significant stenosis generally have a similar color throughout the lumen of the vessel; however, there may be alterations of color associated with the cardiac cycle in nonstenotic vessels. Eddy effects may be also present in regions of vessel dilation in the absence of stenosis. Taking the time to adjust the color Doppler settings appropriately facilitates stenosis detection, because aliasing is likely present in a significant stenosis. If a stenosis is suspected on color imaging, it needs to be visually verified with gray scale for luminal narrowing, and spectral Doppler used to analyze velocities.

For spectral Doppler evaluation, the Doppler cursor angle should be parallel to the posterior vessel wall with an angle of 60° or less; the gate should be within the center of the vessel. If a stenosis is present, the angle of evaluation should be changed from parallel to the posterior vessel wall to parallel to the jet seen at or distal to the stenosis. Several Doppler samples may be required to find the maximum peak systolic velocity (PSV) in a jet associated with a stenosis.

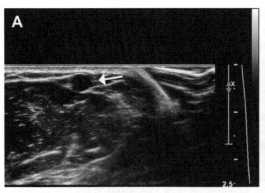
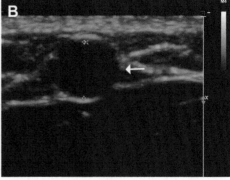

Fig. 2. Gray-scale imaging. (*A*) Transverse gray-scale image of the mid upper arm cephalic vein (*arrow*) with suboptimal field of view resulting in many wasted pixels using a lower-frequency 12-MHz linear transducer. (*B*) Transverse gray-scale image of the mid upper arm cephalic vein shows optimal field of view, focal zone placement, and a round noncompressed vessel (*arrow*). A higher-frequency linear transducer 15 MHz was used. Proper technique permits better assessment of luminal diameter.

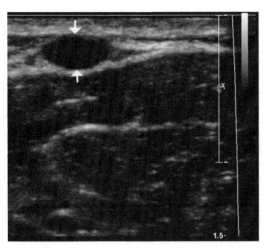

Fig. 3. Manual compression from probe deforms venous wall (*arrows*) and results in suboptimal measurement.

Heel-toe manipulation of the transducer may be required to keep the Doppler angle of insonation less than 60°, if the angle cannot be steered adequately. Baseline and Doppler pulse repetition frequency settings may have to be changed to keep the Doppler waveform within approximately 75% of the velocity scale window without aliasing (**Fig. 6**). The spectral Doppler gain should be adjusted to adequately reflect the velocity profile without excessive background noise and loss of the spectral window in a nonturbulent vessel (gain set too high) or loss of the highest velocities in the waveform (gain set too low). The wall filter should be adjusted for the vessel evaluated as follows: low for slow venous flow and medium to high for an artery or arterialized access.

Blood Flow (Volume Flow) Measurement

Blood flow can be measured in the brachial artery, draining vein of the fistula or graft, and within the graft in mL/min, using the volume flow measurement function on the ultrasound scanner. Careful technique is crucial when measuring blood flow, because there are many potential pitfalls of this measurement, and errors can easily attain 10% to 20%.[28,29] The highest-frequency transducer available that gives optimal lumen definition should be used, with the focal zone centered at the vessel.[28] Abundant gel, beam steering, and potential heel-toe angulation of the transducer should be used to achieve a 60° angle of insonation relative to the back wall of the artery.

The Doppler sample volume (gate) is adjusted to encompass the entire vessel width without extending significantly past the walls. This gate width is different from that routinely used for other spectral Doppler imaging. The velocity spectrum should be adjusted to encompass approximately 75% of the spectral window, and the baseline should be adjusted to avoid aliasing, as discussed earlier. At least 3 spectral cardiac cycles from the Doppler tracing should be evaluated in the time-averaged mean velocity calculation. The internal vessel diameter measurement should be placed perpendicular to the back wall of the vessel and include only the intraluminal diameter. The ultrasound scanner then calculates the blood flow as time-averaged mean velocity multiplied by the area of the vessel (**Fig. 7**).

Stenosis Evaluation

Spectral Doppler vessel evaluation for arteries, grafts, or veins should be performed 2 cm upstream from the stenosis and at the stenosis (or distal jet) to allow calculation of the PSV ratio. If the velocity jet is not parallel to the back wall of the vessel then angle correction should be performed to the angle of the color jet, keeping the Doppler angle less than or equal to 60°. PSV and end diastolic velocity (EDV) are measured at

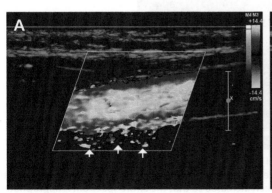
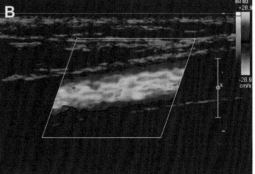

Fig. 4. Color Doppler imaging. (*A*) Color bleed (*arrows*) is present when color pixels extend into the tissue outside the brachial artery wall. Color scale is at 14.4 cm/s. (*B*) Increasing the color scale to 28.9 cm/s (*upper right*) yields an optimal image. Color fills the lumen of the brachial artery without extension beyond the vessel wall.

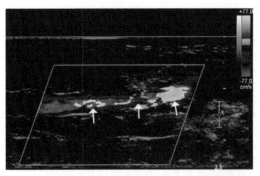

Fig. 5. Color Doppler aliasing. Aliasing (*arrows*) at a stenosis in the draining vein of an upper arm fistula. Central luminal flow that would normally be depicted as red to light orange is displayed as light blue and dark blue because of the focally increased velocity at the stenosis.

each site. The location of the stenosis in relation to the closest anastomosis is recorded (**Fig. 8**). A gray-scale longitudinal image of the stenosis is obtained so the visual degree of narrowing may be evaluated (**Fig. 9**). A juxta-anastomotic fistula stenosis is characterized by the following criteria at our institution: (1) within 2 cm of the anastomosis, encompassing both feeding artery and draining vein[30,31]; (2) having a PSV ratio of greater than or equal to 3:1; and (3) showing visible narrowing. An arterial limb stenosis in a graft is characterized by a PSV ratio greater than or equal to 3:1 and visible narrowing. Draining vein, venous limb, and intragraft stenoses are characterized by a PSV ratio greater than or equal to 2:1 and visible narrowing (**Table 1**).

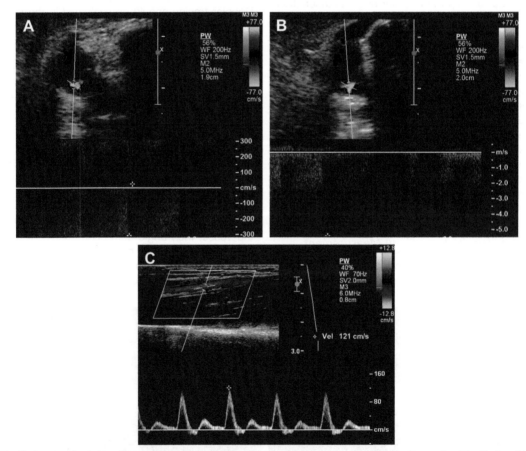

Fig. 6. Spectral Doppler aliasing. (*A*) Suboptimal spectral Doppler image of an AVF anastomosis with aliasing. The velocity scale should be adjusted and the baseline moved to 1 end of the scale. (*B*) The velocity range has been increased from 0.6 m/s to 5.0 m/s and the baseline has been increased so that the entire spectrum is appropriately displayed. (*C*) Optimal spectral Doppler image with 60° angle, gate parallel to back wall of the vessel, and gate within center of vessel. PSV 121.0 cm/s. Note the normal biphasic waveform of the brachial artery from this planning ultrasound scan.

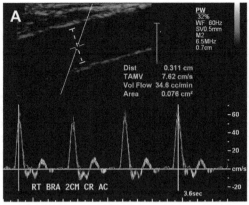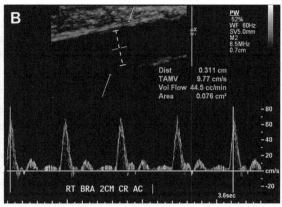

Fig. 7. Blood flow brachial artery. (*A*) Suboptimal blood flow image because the Doppler gate does not include the entire vessel lumen and only 2 cardiac cycles are included. Volume flow is calculated at 34.6 mL/min. (*B*) Optimal blood flow image. The Doppler angle is 60° and parallel with the back wall; the gate is open to include the vessel diameter and 3 cardiac waveforms are included. Luminal diameter is measured with paddles immediately adjacent to the intima. The correct volume flow is calculated at 44.5 mL/min.

HEMODIALYSIS ACCESS PLANNING ULTRASOUND SCAN

An arteriovenous fistula should be placed when clinically appropriate, and whenever anatomically possible. Access placement into the nondominant arm is preferable over the dominant arm, so activities of daily living can be performed while the nondominant arm heals. However, a dominant arm fistula is preferred over a nondominant graft. Potential access sites in decreasing order of preference are as follows: a forearm AVF (radiocephalic AVF, or transposed forearm basilic vein to radial artery), an upper arm brachiocephalic AVF or transposed brachiobasilic AVF, a forearm loop graft, an upper arm straight graft (brachial artery to upper basilic vein), an upper arm axillary artery to axillary vein loop graft, and a thigh graft. Cephalic vein AVFs are preferred over transposition AVFs because less dissection and vein handling are required. Other less common access configurations are also possible based on surgical experience.[32,33]

The preoperative criteria used at our institution include a minimum intraluminal arterial diameter of 2.0 mm and a minimal intraluminal venous diameter of 2.5 mm for AVF.[6,11] For graft creation, a minimum intraluminal venous diameter of 4.0 mm is used, with the same arterial diameter threshold of 2.0 mm as used in AVFs.[6]

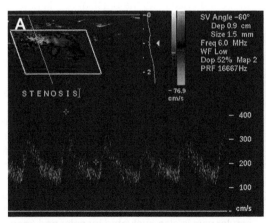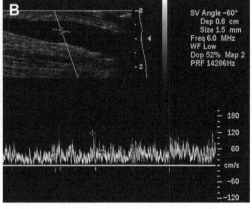

Fig. 8. Spectral Doppler AVF draining vein stenosis. (*A*) Spectral Doppler at stenosis located in the draining vein of an AVF at 4 cm cranial to anastomosis with PSV 414.4 cm/s. Doppler cursor is placed in the area of aliasing. (*B*) Spectral Doppler 2 cm cranial to anastomosis (2 cm caudal [upstream]) from draining vein stenosis with PSV 118.4 cm/s. Given the PSV in (*A*), this process yields a PSV ratio of 3.5:1.

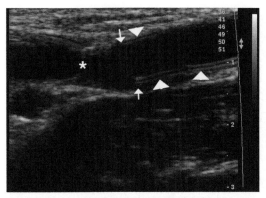

Fig. 9. Graft stenosis. Longitudinal gray-scale image shows luminal narrowing (*asterisk*) beyond the venous to graft anastomosis. Arrows mark the venous anastomosis. The graft wall is identified by its parallel echogenic lines (*arrowheads*).

Arterial Evaluation

The lower third of the brachial and radial arteries should be assessed for intimal thickening, calcification, stenosis or occlusion using gray-scale imaging in the transverse and longitudinal planes. If a parvus tardus waveform (a small-amplitude waveform with a prolonged systolic increase) is noted, a more proximal evaluation of the artery may be necessary to evaluate for proximal stenosis. Calcifications may be categorized as absent, mild to moderate, or severe (**Fig. 10**). A brachial artery intraluminal diameter is obtained in the transverse plane 2 cm cranial to the antecubital fossa, and the radial artery is assessed 2 cm cranial to the wrist. Color and spectral Doppler should be performed in the longitudinal plane at the same location. Peak systolic velocities are measured, and the waveforms are inspected for normal triphasic or biphasic flow (**Fig. 11**).

If 2 arteries are visualized with accompanying paired veins in the upper arm, a high radial artery takeoff from the brachial artery should be

Table 1 Access stenoses	
Stenosis Type	**Stenosis Criteria**
AVF: juxta-anastomotic (within 2 cm of the anastomosis)	PSV ratio ≥3:1 Visible narrowing
Graft: arterial-graft anastomosis	PSV ratio ≥3:1 Visible narrowing
Graft: venous-graft anastomosis, intragraft stenosis	PSV ratio ≥2:1 Visible narrowing
AVF or graft: feeding artery, draining vein	PSV ratio ≥2:1 Visible narrowing

suspected (**Fig. 12**). Both arteries should be followed into the forearm to distinguish this common anatomic variant from a prominent arterial branch to the elbow region.

Venous Assessment

A tourniquet should be sequentially placed before evaluation of the upper extremity veins first in the mid forearm to image the cephalic vein from the wrist to mid forearm, second just above the antecubital fossa to image veins of the mid forearm to cranial forearm and antecubital fossa, and subsequently in the axillary/upper arm area to image the upper arm veins.[34] Venous assessment is performed after arterial assessment, because application of a tourniquet may alter arterial blood flow and waveforms.

Veins should be assessed with visual inspection and compression along their length. Venous diameters should be measured in the transverse plane using gray-scale imaging from anterior wall intima to posterior wall intima for an intraluminal diameter. Cephalic vein diameters are measured in the caudal, mid, and cranial aspects of the forearm and upper arm with distance from the skin to the lumen of the anterior (superficial) venous wall recorded (**Fig. 13**). Basilic vein diameters are measured at the antecubital fossa and the caudal, mid, and cranial upper arm. The basilic vein diameter is also measured at 4 cm caudal to the antecubital fossa to assess the diameter of the additional vein length needed for the brachiobasilic transposition fistula. The basilic vein must be transposed and placed more superficially in the soft tissues; thus basilic vein to skin depth is not measured. The length of the upper arm basilic vein before joining with the brachial veins does not usually alter the planned surgery, but the location where it empties into the brachial vein is noted for the surgeon's information.

The tourniquet is removed and the cephalic vein is followed centrally to ensure that it empties into the deep venous system. The axillary vein diameter is recorded. Occasionally, overlying muscle may cause a stenotic appearance at the cephalic vein insertion into the subclavian vein junction that is accentuated by abduction; adducting the arm may alleviate an apparent stenosis at this point. The patient is placed in the supine position for optimal assessment of the subclavian and internal jugular veins. The cranial and caudal aspects of the internal jugular vein are assessed by manual compression to exclude thrombus. The internal jugular vein is also evaluated by color and spectral Doppler to evaluate for transmitted cardiac pulsatility and respiratory phasicity, indirect signs of normal flow. The medial and lateral subclavian

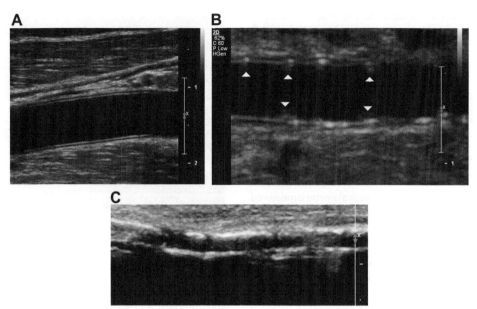

Fig. 10. Arterial calcification assessment. (*A*) Brachial artery with no calcifications. (*B*) Magnified image of radial artery with mild calcification (*arrowheads*). (*C*) Radial artery with severe calcification in extended view.

veins are also evaluated with color and spectral Doppler to assess for transmitted cardiac pulsatility and respiratory phasicity (**Fig. 14**). If either vein does not show normal transmitted cardiac pulsatility or respiratory phasicity, further evaluation while the patient performs Valsalva or the sniff test may reveal a normal waveform that returns to baseline.

HEMODIALYSIS ACCESS ASSESSMENT ULTRASOUND SCAN

Many of the basic principles and techniques of the access planning ultrasound scan can be used in the evaluation of an existing access, with some modifications as described later. An initial overview of the access is obtained from patient history, operative notes, and initial scan. The caudal third of the feeding artery is assessed in the transverse plane using gray scale to evaluate for stenosis. The intraluminal diameter of the feeding artery is measured 2 cm cranial (upstream) to the anastomosis. Color and spectral Doppler are performed in the longitudinal plane at the same location. PSV and EDV are measured, and the waveform is inspected for normal monophasic (low-resistance) flow (**Fig. 15**). If the patient has symptoms of arterial steal, such as pain during or off dialysis or less frequently loss of distal function, the arterial flow to the hand should be evaluated downstream to the anastomosis. Reversal of flow in the artery distal to the anastomosis is consistent with steal, although it is frequently asymptomatic. Gentle transient compression of the AVF or graft while

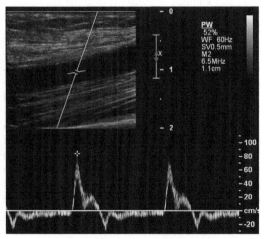

Fig. 11. Spectral Doppler image of the brachial artery shows a normal biphasic waveform (triphasic is normal as well).

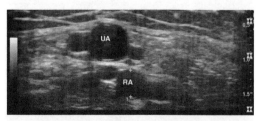

Fig. 12. High bifurcation of the brachial artery should be suspected when 2 arteries are identified near the antecubital fossa. The radial artery (RA) is denoted by calipers and the ulnar artery (UA) is anterior to it.

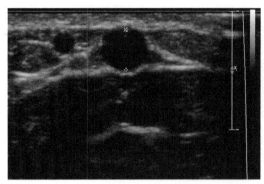

Fig. 13. Mid forearm cephalic vein diameter is measured in a transverse gray-scale image. Crosshairs (+) abut the internal margins of the anterior and posterior venous walls for luminal diameter measurement. Distance from skin surface to anterior wall lumen (x) is measured to show depth for access. Vessels greater than 5 mm from the skin surface are often difficult to cannulate.

measuring the spectral waveform in the distal artery usually shows a return to normal antegrade high-resistance flow in the distal artery, confirming the diagnosis.

Anastomoses

AVF

The arteriovenous anastomosis is evaluated with gray scale in transverse and longitudinal planes to assess for stenosis or thrombosis. Color and spectral Doppler are then performed in the longitudinal plane of the artery 2 cm cranial to the anastomosis, and in the anastomotic region extending into the draining vein at the anastomosis. Proper placement of the gate and Doppler angle during spectral Doppler is important to achieve accurate

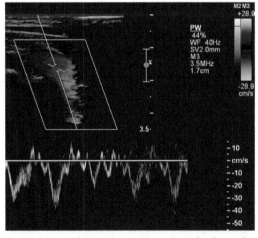

Fig. 14. Spectral Doppler images show both cardiac pulsatility and respiratory phasicity in the right medial subclavian vein.

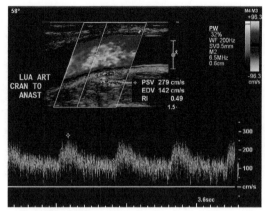

Fig. 15. Spectral Doppler image of the brachial artery 2 cm cranial to the anastomosis shows a normal low-resistance waveform. PSV 279 cm/s. EDV 142 cm/s.

measurements of the highest velocity within the anastomosis, as described earlier. PSV and EDV are measured at both locations. At our institution we define a juxta-anastomotic stenosis as within 2 cm of the anastomosis, which includes both feeding artery and draining vein (see **Table 1**).[30,31]

Grafts

After evaluation of the feeding artery, the arterial anastomosis of a graft is assessed with color and spectral Doppler, with PSV and EDV measured in the same way as for a fistula. Additional spectral waveform PSV and EDV are measured 2 cm upstream to the venous anastomosis within the graft and at the venous anastomosis. A spectral waveform is also obtained within the mid portion of the graft in a straight graft, and both the arterial and venous limbs of a loop graft. If the graft is thrombosed, a longitudinal gray-scale image is obtained to show intraluminal thrombus. Color and spectral Doppler images are obtained to verify the lack of flow.

Draining Vein

In an AVF or graft, the entire draining vein is assessed visually for wall thickening, stenosis, and thrombosis with gray-scale imaging in the transverse plane throughout its length. In a fistula, the intraluminal vein diameter and the distance from skin surface are measured in the transverse plane using gray scale at multiple points cranial to the AVF anastomosis. The vein is measured in the caudal, mid, and upper forearm and in the upper arm for a forearm AVF, and in the caudal, mid, and cranial upper arm for an upper arm fistula. The draining vein is evaluated for accessory vein branches in the first 10 to 15 cm cranial to the anastomosis. If such branches are identified, the size and distance from the anastomosis are recorded for each vessel (**Fig. 16**). The draining vein in the upper arm is similarly evaluated for a forearm graft, and the remaining basilic/axillary vein is evaluated for an upper arm graft. The subclavian and internal jugular veins do not need to be evaluated routinely, because they were already assessed preoperatively, except in patients with arm swelling in whom a more central obstruction may be present.

Three flow volume measurements are obtained within the graft or mid draining vein of an AVF in an area with parallel walls without vessel tortuosity or stenosis. Several pilot studies suggest that blood flow rates increase within minutes to days after AVF creation, and early flow rates may be useful in differentiating between AVFs that eventually mature and those that fail.[10,35,36] Grafts with decreased blood flow have been shown to be at an increased risk for thrombosis.[18,37,38] The presence of fluid collections should be noted; when present these are measured and inspected for echogenic foci or gas. If the access is thrombosed, this is further documented with color and spectral Doppler. Power Doppler may be more sensitive for detection of residual slow flow.

DIAGNOSTIC CRITERIA
Arteriovenous Fistulas

Normal AVF findings
The typical sonographic findings of a normal AVF are antegrade flow throughout the arterial (see **Fig. 15**) and venous limbs (**Fig. 17**) without visible narrowing or flow disturbance. Color and spectral Doppler imaging show no focal increased velocity or aliasing to suggest stenosis. The average volumetric flow in functioning AVFs is at least 300 to 800 mL/min.[10,18,39,40] We correlated sonographic fistula measurements with clinically determined

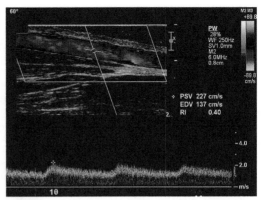

Fig. 17. Color Doppler shows antegrade flow and smooth color within the draining vein without aliasing or turbulence.

maturation, and found that about 70% of AVFs could be used for hemodialysis with a minimum draining vein of 4 mm or greater or a blood flow rate of 500 mL/min or greater.[10] If both criteria were present, the likelihood of fistula maturation was 95%. Only 33% of fistulas were adequate for hemodialysis if neither criterion was met. The National Kidney Foundation Kidney Disease Outcomes Quality Initiative (DOQI) recently published sonographic criteria suggestive of fistula maturation. These criteria include a draining vein diameter of greater than 6 mm, venous outflow of at least 600 mL/min, and a distance of less than 6 mm from the skin surface as predictors of successful maturation.[3] However, if the higher DOQI criterion were applied to our patient population, the number of fistulas that were suitable for hemodialysis was underestimated by 30% (Michael Allon, personal communication, 2011).

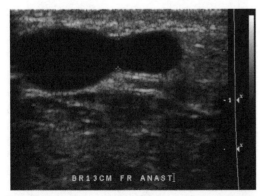

Fig. 16. Transverse gray-scale image depicts a venous branch emanating from the AVF draining vein. Calipers denote the origin of the branch and its size (0.32 cm in this case). The distance of the branch from the anastomosis (13 cm) is also annotated on the image.

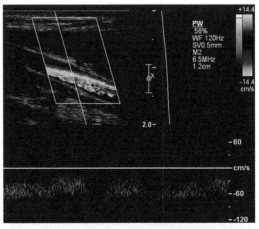

Fig. 18. Spectral Doppler shows monophasic flow in the internal jugular vein, suggesting proximal thrombosis or stenosis. Compare with the normal pulsatile flow in **Fig. 14**.

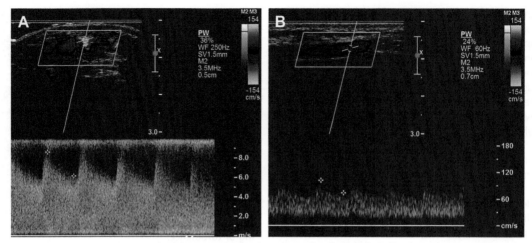

Fig. 19. Juxta-anastomotic stenosis. (A) Spectral Doppler image shows turbulent flow and increased PSV of 861 cm/s at the juxta-anastomotic stenosis. (B) Spectral Doppler image of feeding artery 2 cm upstream from anastomosis with PSV 102 cm/s, which yields a PSV ratio of 8.4.

The brachiocephalic veins are indirectly assessed by Doppler imaging of the internal jugular and subclavian veins. Spectral Doppler assessment of normal central veins shows signs of respiratory phasicity and transmitted cardiac pulsatility. Monophasic subclavian and internal jugular venous waveforms suggest a central venous stenosis or occlusion (Fig. 18).

ABNORMALITIES

AVF abnormalities include stenosis, thrombosis, pseudoaneurysm, arterial steal, and perifistula fluid collections. Findings of stenosis include visual narrowing on gray-scale imaging and an increased PSV ratio at the site of stenosis relative to the vessel 2 cm upstream. We use a PSV ratio of

3:1 for diagnosis of juxta-anastomotic stenosis of 50% or greater (Fig. 19) and a ratio of 2:1 for draining vein stenosis of 50% or greater (see Fig. 8). Arterial inflow stenoses are rare but do occur and are also diagnosed by a PSV ratio of 2:1 for a 50% or greater stenosis. Stenoses are most common in the juxta-anastomotic region, followed by the draining vein, and then central veins.[14] They are clinically relevant because stenoses within AVFs may be associated with subsequent thrombosis. The diagnosis of thrombosis is made when no flow is identified within the AVF. Thrombus is usually visualized within the lumen on gray-scale imaging (Fig. 20). Power Doppler

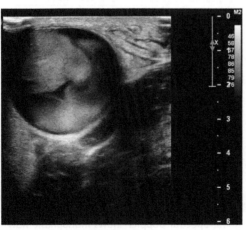

Fig. 20. Occluded AVF. Gray-scale transverse image shows occlusive echogenic thrombus within the draining vein of the AVF.

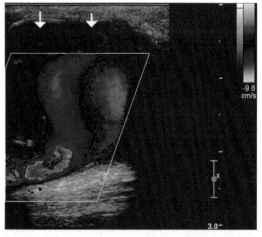

Fig. 21. Color Doppler image shows the typical bidirectional blue and red (yin-yang) flow pattern of a pseudoaneurysm (arrows). Marginal thrombus prevents flow from completely filling the lumen.

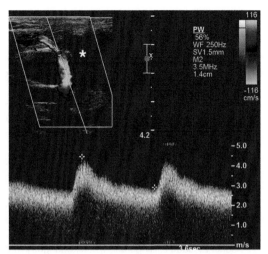

Fig. 22. Spectral Doppler image shows a hypoechoic fluid collection (*asterisk*) compressing the draining vein of an AVF, resulting in increased velocities.

can be used to exclude slow flow. Pseudoaneurysms usually develop from suboptimal compression after cannulation. A pseudoaneurysm is well evaluated by color Doppler, showing a typical yin/yang pattern (**Fig. 21**), which represents blood flowing into and then out of the focal defect in the fistula wall. Avascular, perifistula hypoechoic fluid collections are commonly seen, and usually represent postaccess or procedure hematomas (**Fig. 22**). Echogenic foci with shadowing within a fluid collection may represent gas, suggestive of infection, in the correct clinical setting.

Arteriovenous Grafts

Synthetic grafts made of polytetrafluoroethylene are easily identified sonographically by 2 characteristic echogenic lines representing a strong specular reflection from the graft material.

NORMAL GRAFT FINDINGS

Normal graft findings at ultrasonography include antegrade arterialized flow without focal turbulence, visible narrowing, or focally increased velocity. Graft waveforms are monophasic with a low-resistance arterialized waveform. Draining venous flow should be antegrade without focal turbulence or aliasing. Because of the larger volume of flow in grafts, the absence of phasicity in the central veins is less specific for central occlusion than for fistulas.

Graft Abnormalities

Common graft abnormalities are similar to those of AVF and include stenosis, thrombosis, and pseudoaneurysm, as well as graft degeneration and arterial steal. As mentioned earlier, grafts with decreased blood flow are at increased risk for thrombosis according to several studies.[10,18,37,38] Graft stenosis is characterized by 3 sonographic criteria: (1) visual luminal narrowing on gray-scale imaging, (2) a high-velocity jet on color Doppler, and (3) a PSV ratio greater than 2:1 (venous anastomotic or draining vein) or 3:1 (arterial anastomosis), as described earlier. The most common sites of graft stenosis are in decreasing order of prevalence as follows: venous anastomosis, draining vein, intragraft, arterial anastomosis, and central veins.[10] The diagnosis of thrombosis is made when no flow is identified within the graft. Thrombus is usually visualized as mildly echogenic material within the lumen on gray-scale imaging. Power Doppler can be used to exclude slow flow.

Pseudoaneurysm formation is relatively common and is characterized by the typical yin/yang flow pattern with color Doppler. Graft degeneration can be diagnosed with depiction of a very irregular graft wall, and may be associated with

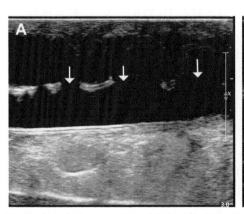

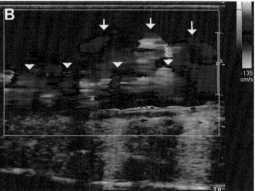

Fig. 23. Graft wall degeneration. (*A*) Gray-scale image shows irregularity (*arrows*) of the graft wall most prominent along the anterior wall. Arrows denote foci of graft wall degeneration. (*B*) Color Doppler image indicates several pseudoaneurysms (*arrows*) protruding beyond the expected location of the wall (*arrowheads*).

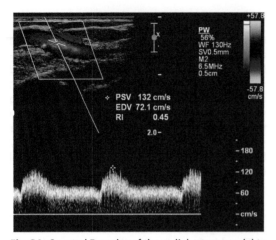

Fig. 24. Spectral Doppler of the radial artery caudal to the anastomosis shows reversal of flow (arterial flow heading toward the transducer, thus away from the fingers and toward the heart) consistent with arterial steal. Note the abnormal low-resistance waveform.

numerous pseudoaneurysms along the course of the graft (**Fig. 23**). Arterial steal, defined as flow reversal in the native artery caudal to the anastomosis, is commonly seen and may be symptomatic (**Fig. 24**). Symptoms include hand pain and burning that worsen during dialysis. Ischemia or frank necrosis of the fingers may occur. Arterial steal was reported in 24% of patients with grafts in 1 series, all of whom were asymptomatic.[41] Sonographic evaluation shows reversal of flow in the distal radial artery and rarely shows an occluded artery. Brief manual compression of the graft usually shows radial artery flow reversal with an antegrade high-resistance flow pattern toward the hand.

SUMMARY

Ultrasonography can significantly improve access planning, and postoperative fistula and graft evaluation in the hemodialysis patient. Careful sonographic technique with knowledge of anatomy and common and uncommon access abnormalities results in a thorough and accurate evaluation.

REFERENCES

1. U.S. Renal Data System, USRDS 2010 Annual Data Report. Atlas of chronic kidney disease and end-stage renal disease in the United States. Bethesda (MD): National Institutes of Health, National Institute of Diabetes and Digestive and Kidney Diseases; 2010.
2. Feldman HI, Kobrin S, Wasserstein A. Hemodialysis vascular access morbidity. J Am Soc Nephrol 1996; 7:523–35.
3. KDOQI clinical practice guidelines and clinical practice recommendations for vascular access 2006. Am J Kidney Dis 2006;48(Suppl 1):S176–322.
4. Hodges TC, Fillinger MF, Zwolak RM, et al. Longitudinal comparison of dialysis access methods: risk factors for failure. J Vasc Surg 1997;26:1009–19.
5. Stevenson KB, Hannah EL, Lowder CA, et al. Epidemiology of hemodialysis vascular access infections from longitudinal infection surveillance data: predicting the impact of NKF-DOQI clinical practice guidelines for vascular access. Am J Kidney Dis 2002;39: 549–55.
6. Silva MB Jr, Hobson RW 2nd, Pappas PJ, et al. A strategy for increasing use of autogenous hemodialysis access procedures: impact of preoperative noninvasive evaluation. J Vasc Surg 1998;27:302–7.
7. Ascher E, Gade P, Hingorani A, et al. Changes in the practice of angioaccess surgery: impact of dialysis outcome and quality initiative recommendations. J Vasc Surg 2000;31:84–92.
8. Gibson KD, Caps MT, Kohler TR, et al. Assessment of a policy to reduce placement of prosthetic hemodialysis access. Kidney Int 2001;59:2335–45.
9. Allon M, Lockhart ME, Lilly RZ, et al. Effect of preoperative sonographic mapping on vascular access outcomes in hemodialysis patients. Kidney Int 2001;60:2013–20.
10. Robbin ML, Chamberlain NE, Lockhart ME, et al. Hemodialysis arteriovenous fistula maturity: US evaluation. Radiology 2002;225:59–64.
11. Robbin ML, Gallichio MH, Deierhoi MH, et al. US vascular mapping before hemodialysis access placement. Radiology 2000;217:83–8.
12. Besarab A, Sullivan KL, Ross RP, et al. Utility of intra-access pressure monitoring in detecting and correcting venous outlet stenoses before thrombosis. Kidney Int 1995;47:1364–73.
13. Schwab SJ, Raymond JR, Saeed M, et al. Prevention of hemodialysis fistula thrombosis: early detection of venous stenoses. Kidney Int 1989;36:707–11.
14. Beuter JJ, Lezanna AH, Calvo JH, et al. Early detection and treatment of hemodialysis access dysfunction. Cardiovasc Intervent Radiol 2000;23:40–6.
15. Sands J, Young S, Miranda C. The effect of Doppler flow screening studies and elective revisions on dialysis access failure. ASAIO J 1992;38:M524–7.
16. Safa AA, Valji K, Roberts AC, et al. Detection and treatment of dysfunctional hemodialysis access grafts: effects of a surveillance program on graft patency and the incidence of thrombosis. Radiology 1996;199:653–7.
17. Allon M, Bailey R, Ballard R, et al. A multidisciplinary approach to hemodialysis access: prospective evaluation. Kidney Int 1998;53:473–9.
18. Bay WH, Henry ML, Lazarus JM, et al. Predicting hemodialysis access failure with color Doppler ultrasound. Am J Nephrol 1998;18:296–304.

19. Robbin ML, Oser RF, Lee JY, et al. Randomized comparison of ultrasound surveillance and clinical monitoring on arteriovenous graft outcomes. Kidney Int 2006;69:730–5.

20. Lumsden AB, MacDonald MJ, Kikeri D, et al. Prophylactic balloon angioplasty fails to prolong the patency of expanded polytetrafluoroethylene arteriovenous grafts: results of a prospective randomized study. J Vasc Surg 1997;26:382–92.

21. Ram SJ, Work J, Caldito GC, et al. A randomized controlled trial of blood flow and stenosis surveillance of hemodialysis grafts. Kidney Int 2003;64:272–80.

22. Malik J, Slavikova M, Svobodova J, et al. Regular ultrasound screening significantly prolongs patency of grafts. Kidney Int 2005;67:1554–8.

23. Dember LM, Holmberg EF, Kaufman JS. Randomized controlled trial of prophylactic repair of hemodialysis arteriovenous graft stenosis. Kidney Int 2004; 66:390–8.

24. Singh P, Robbin ML, Lockhart ME, et al. Clinically immature arteriovenous hemodialysis fistulas: effect of US on salvage. Radiology 2008;246:299–305.

25. Asif A, Roy-Chadhury P, Beathard GA. Early arteriovenous fistula failure: a logical proposal for how and when to intervene. Clin J Am Soc Nephrol 2006;1:332–9.

26. Robbin ML, Osler RF, Allon M, et al. Hemodialysis access graft stenosis: US detection. Radiology 1998;208:655–61.

27. Lockhart ME, Robbin ML. Hemodialysis ultrasound. Ultrasound Q 2001;17:157–67.

28. Hoyt K, Hester F, Bell R, et al. Accuracy of volumetric flow rate measurements–an in vitro study using modern US scanners. J Ultrasound Med 2009;28:1511–8.

29. Winkler AJ, Wu J, Case T, et al. An experimental study of the accuracy of volume flow measurements using commercial ultrasound systems. J Vasc Tech 1995;19:175–80.

30. Clark TW, Hirsch DA, Jindal KJ, et al. Outcome and prognostic factors of restenosis after percutaneous treatment of native hemodialysis fistulas. J Vasc Interv Radiol 2002;13:51–9.

31. Beathard GA, Arnold P, Jackson J, et al. Aggressive treatment of early fistula failure. Physician Operators Forum of RMS Lifeline. Kidney Int 2003;64:1487–94.

32. Jennings WC, Sideman MJ, Taubman KE, et al. Brachial vein transposition arteriovenous fistulas for hemodialysis access. J Vasc Surg 2009;50: 1121–5.

33. Jennings WC. Creating arteriovenous fistulas in 132 consecutive patients: exploiting the proximal radial artery arteriovenous fistula: reliable, safe, and simple forearm and upper arm hemodialysis access. Arch Surg 2006;141:27–32.

34. Lockhart ME, Robbin ML, Fineberg NS, et al. Cephalic vein measurement before forearm fistula creation: does use of a tourniquet to meet venous diameter threshold increase the number of useable fistulas? J Ultrasound Med 2006;25:1541–5.

35. Won T, Jang JW, Lee S, et al. Effects of intraoperative blood flow on the early patency of radiocephalic fistulas. Ann Vasc Surg 2000;14:468–72.

36. Corpataux JM, Haesler E, Silacci P, et al. Low-pressure environment and remodelling of the forearm vein in Brescia-Cimino haemodialysis access. Nephrol Dial Transplant 2002;17:1057–62.

37. May RE, Himmelfarb J, Yenicesu M, et al. Predictive measures of vascular access thrombosis: a prospective study. Kidney Int 1997;52:1656–62.

38. Shackleton CR, Taylor DC, Buckely AR, et al. Predicting failure in polytetrafluoroethylene vascular access grafts for hemodialysis: a pilot study. Can J Surg 1987;30:442–4.

39. Falk A. Maintenance and salvage of arteriovenous fistulas. J Vasc Interv Radiol 2006;17:807–13.

40. Back MR, Maynard M, Winkler A, et al. Expected flow parameters within hemodialysis access and selection for remedial intervention of nonmaturing conduits. Vasc Endovascular Surg 2008;42:150–8.

41. Valji K, Hye RJ, Roberts AC, et al. Hand ischemia in patients with hemodialysis access grafts: angiographic diagnosis and treatment. Radiology 1995; 196:697–701.

Ultrasound Evaluation of Renovascular Hypertension

Steven Y. Wang, MD*, Leslie M. Scoutt, MD

KEYWORDS

• Ultrasound • Renovascular hypertension

Hypertension is an increasingly prevalent condition, now affecting 29% of Americans.[1] Most patients with hypertension have no identifiable cause and are considered to have essential hypertension. Renovascular hypertension, or hypertension caused by renal artery stenosis, is rare and is estimated to account for less than 1% to 3% of all hypertensive cases.[2] However, renovascular hypertension is the most common surgically treatable cause of hypertension and, if untreated, the end result may be renal failure. In 1934, Goldblatt and colleagues[3] first showed that reduction in perfusion to even 1 kidney could induce sustained hypertension. It has subsequently been shown that decreased renal perfusion leads to activation of the renin-angiotension-aldosterone cascade, which ultimately triggers the development of hypertension. In addition, recently published data suggest that angiotensin activates other downstream pressor mechanisms involving the endothelium, myocardium, and sympathetic nerves.[2,4]

EPIDEMIOLOGY AND THERAPY

In the United States, atherosclerosis, or more generally termed atherosclerotic renovascular disease (ARVD), is the underlying pathology in over 90% of patients with renovascular hypertension (RVH). ARVD tends to involve the origins or proximal third of the renal arteries and less commonly branch points. If untreated, ARVD can lead to acceleration of pre-existing HT, renal insufficiency, congestive heart failure, pulmonary edema, hypertensive encephalopathy, stroke, and aortic aneurysm. It is believed that ARVD accounts for approximately 15% of cases of chronic renal failure.[5] The prevalence of ARVD increases with age, reaching as high as 6.8% in 1 study of patients 65 years of age and older.[6] Studies have shown that 13% of patients with pre-existing ARVD in 1 renal artery can progress to hemodynamically significant stenosis in the remaining normal renal artery within 3 years.[7,8] It is estimated that less than 20% of stenotic arteries will progress to complete occlusion.[7–11] Thus the task for clinicians is to detect the RVH due to ARVD as well as halt its progression before irreversible damage is done to the kidneys.

Treatment of ARVD has traditionally focused on revascularization, either with surgical by-pass grafts or with percutaneous angioplasty or stenting. Percutaneous balloon renal angioplasty was introduced in the 1990s. However, technical success rates were initially reported to be relatively low at 50% to 62%, and the restenosis rate is reportedly as high as 47% in some series.[12] More recently, the introduction of intravascular stents has vastly improved technical success rates to near 100%, and restenosis rates have been reported to be much lower, ranging from 0% to 23%.[12] In recent years, the topic of revascularization for treatment of ARVD has become increasingly controversial. Three small randomized–controlled trials, although underpowered, failed to show clinical benefit of revascularization when compared with optimal medical treatment.[13] Subsequently, a recently reported large randomized control trial performed in the United States demonstrated no clinical benefit from revascularization procedures.[14] Many hypotheses have been put forward as to why revascularization may not help. It is postulated that given

Department of Diagnostic Radiology, Yale University School of Medicine, 333 Cedar Street, PO Box 208042, New Haven, CT 06520-8042, USA
* Corresponding author.
E-mail address: steven.wang@yale.edu

Ultrasound Clin 6 (2011) 491–511
doi:10.1016/j.cult.2011.07.001
1556-858X/11/$ – see front matter © 2011 Elsevier Inc. All rights reserved.

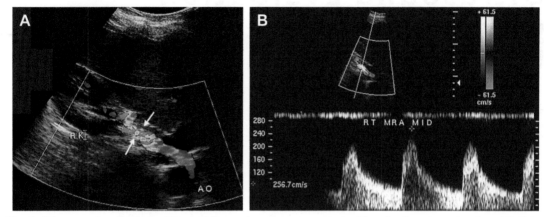

Fig. 1. Fibromuscular dysplasia. This middle-aged woman presented with refractory hypertension. (*A*) Color Doppler ultrasound image demonstrates focal color aliasing (*arrows*) with an irregular or beaded outer wall affecting the middle third of the right main renal artery. (*B*) Spectral Doppler tracing demonstrates a peak systolic velocity (PSV) of 257 cm/s, exceeding the peak systolic velocity threshold for the diagnosis of renal artery stenosis. AO, aorta; RK, right kidney.

the high prevalence of hypertension and athero-sclerosis, atherosclerotic narrowing of the renal artery may simply be an association rather than a causative factor in patients with hypertension. Supporting this idea is the fact that 3% to 7% of normotensive adults can be shown to have inci-dental narrowing of the renal artery by atheroscle-rotic plaque on angiograms performed for other reasons.[15] It is also thought that atherosclerotic stenosis in the renal artery may only be a reflection of underlying intrarenal vascular pathology[16] or that

revascularization does not alter the natural history of the disease, since end-organ damage has already occurred before intervention.[17]

In the United States, fibromuscular dysplasia (FMD) is the underlying cause of RVH in less than 10% of cases. FMD is a disease of unknown etiology that can affect almost any artery, including the carotid, brachial,[18,19] coronary,[20] and pulmo-nary arteries.[21] The renal arteries are involved in 60% to 75% of patients, and the right side is affected twice as often as the left.[5] FMD tends to

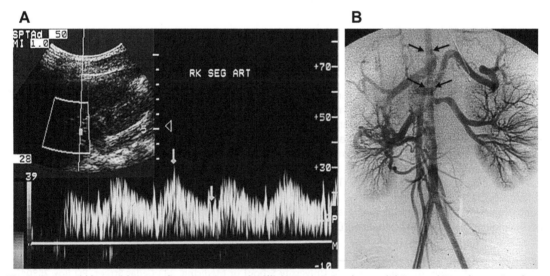

Fig. 2. 8-year-old boy with severe hypertension and William-Beuren Syndrome. (*A*) Spectral Doppler tracing from a segmental artery in the right kidney demonstrates a classic tardus waveform pattern indicative of a proximal stenosis. The intraparenchymal arteries on the left (not shown) demonstrated a similar waveform. (*B*) Angiogram reveals diffuse narrowing of the abdominal aorta (*arrows*) above the origin of the renal arteries. (*Reprinted from Moukaddam H, Pollak J, Scoutt LM. Imaging renal artery stenosis. US Clin 2007;2:468; with permission.*)

cause stenosis of the middle third of the renal artery rather than at the origin, which is the typical location of narrowing due to atherosclerosis. Several pathologic subtypes of FMD have been described. The most common type (75%–80%), medial fibroplasia, produces areas of intima and media thinning, which alternate with regions of media fibrosis, resulting in the classic string-of-beads appearance

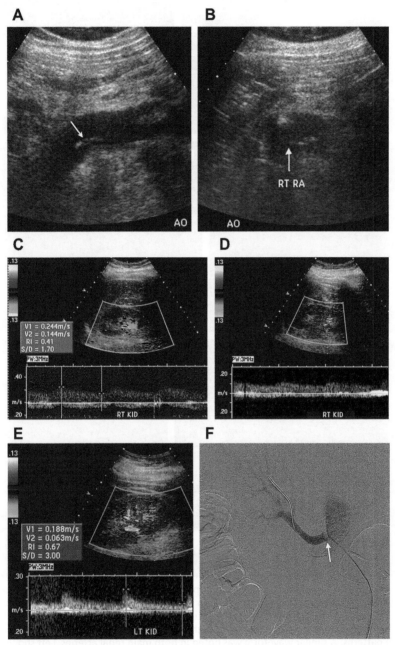

Fig. 3. A 58-year-old man presented with excruciating back pain and hypertension. Sagittal (*A*) and transverse (*B*) images of the aorta demonstrate an echogenic intraluminal flap (*arrow*) from an aortic dissection. On the transverse image (*B*), the dissection flap extended into the origin of the right main artery. Color Doppler image (not shown) revealed that both the true and false lumens were patent. (*C, D*) Spectral Doppler waveforms from segmental arteries in the right kidney demonstrate marked tardus parvus phenomenon. Note slight respiratory variation in the venous waveform below the baseline. (*E*) In comparison, note sharp systolic upstroke in an interlobular arterial waveform from the lower pole of the left kidney. (*F*) Angiogram demonstrates marked narrowing from the dissection flap at the origin of the right main renal artery (*arrow*). The gradient measured 100 mm Hg. The patient was successfully stented resulting in a significant drop in blood pressure. AO, aorta; RA, renal artery.

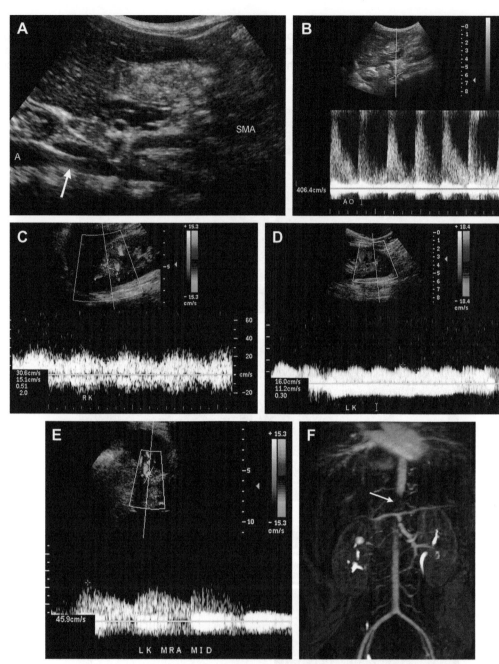

Fig. 4. A 6-year-old boy with neurofibromatosis and upper abdominal aortic coarctation. (*A*) Sagittal gray scale view of the aorta demonstrates narrowing of the lumen (*arrow*) above the origin of the celiac axis and superior mesenteric artery (SMA). (*B*) PSV in the aorta at the level of the narrowing is markedly elevated at 406 cm/s. Spectral waveforms from intraparenchymal vessels in the right (*C*) and left (*D*) kidneys demonstrate bilateral tardus parvus waveform patterns. A similar waveform was noted in both main renal arteries. Left shown (*E*). (*F*) Coronal contrast-enhanced magnetic resonance angiography (MRA) image demonstrates no enhancement (*arrow*) in the markedly narrowed lumen at the site of the upper abdominal aortic coarctation above the origins of the renal arteries. The tardus parvus waveform in the renal arteries is due to the effect of the proximal narrowing (stenosis) of the abdominal aorta and not to bilateral stenoses of the origins renal arteries, which were widely patent.

(Fig. 1).[22] The intimal fibroplasia type is the second most common (5%–10%), and it affects the intima only, resulting in smooth tubular stenoses.[5] Other pathologic subtypes include perimedial fibroplasia and medial hyperplasia.

Most commonly, FMD affects young women in their third to fourth decade of life. Endovascular revascularization is the treatment of choice. Success rates from revascularization procedures are much higher for patients with RVH secondary to FMD than for RVH due to ARVD.[23] Hence, most clinicians agree on the appropriateness of revascularization in this subgroup of patients, although recent work suggests that patients with a nonmedial subtype do not respond as well.[24]

Takayasu arteritis, a chronic granulomatous inflammatory process involving the wall of the aorta and its branches, is a rare cause of RVH in the western world. A study in Minnesota estimated the annual incidence to be 2.6 cases per 1 million population. It is, however, more common in Southeast Asia, South America, and the Mediterranean basin. On the Indian subcontinent, Takayasu arteritis is the most common cause of RVH,[25,26] and bilateral renal involvement is seen in up to 60% of patients.[27] The mainstay of treatment is steroids and other immunosuppressant medications. Revascularization is considered a second-line treatment option.

Williams-Beuren syndrome is a genetic disorder resulting from a defect on the long arm of chromosome 7 (7q11.23), which includes the gene for elastin. In addition to renal artery stenoses contributing to hypertension, this syndrome is also associated with abdominal aortic narrowing, frequently at the level of the renal arteries (Fig. 2).[28] Imaging should also pay attention to renal anomalies, since they are more common in this patient population.[29,30]

Other rare causes of RVH include: vasculitis, radiation injury, renal artery or aortic dissection (Fig. 3), embolization, extrinsic compression by a mass (neurofibromatosis), or middle aortic syndrome. Middle aortic syndrome is the general term for segmental narrowing at the distal descending thoracic aorta or abdominal aorta, which may be due to a congenital coarctation of the aorta, or acquired secondarily through another process such as FMD, Takayasu arteritis, neurofibromatosis (Fig. 4), or Williams-Beuren syndrome.[31,32]

The high prevalence of HT and relative rarity of RVH makes screening of the entire hypertensive population for RVH both impractical and cost-prohibitive. Screening is, therefore, usually reserved for a smaller, enriched subpopulation with significant risk factors for RVH such as those summarized in Box 1.

Box 1
Risk factors for renovascular hypertension

Abdominal bruit

Malignant or accelerated hypertension

Significant hypertension (diastolic blood pressure [BP] >110 mm Hg)

Onset of hypertension in a young adult (<35 years of age)

New onset of hypertension after age 50

Sudden onset or worsening hypertension

Refractory hypertension (eg, to triple-drug therapy)

Absence of family history of hypertension

Hypertension in the setting of renal failure

Recurrent flash pulmonary edema

Deterioration of renal function in response to angiotensin-converting enzyme inhibitors

Generalized atherosclerotic occlusive disease with hypertension

Adapted from American College of Radiology. ACR appropriateness criteria: renovascular hypertension. 2009. Available at: http://www.acr.org/Secondary MainMenuCategories/quality_safety/app_criteria/pdf/ExpertPanelonUrologicImaging/RenovascularHypertensionDoc17.aspx. Accessed March 6, 2011; with permission.

DIAGNOSIS

Intra-arterial digital subtraction angiography (DSA) remains the gold standard for diagnosing renovascular hypertension. In addition to showing excellent anatomic detail, pressure gradients can be measured across stenotic lesions to directly determine whether the lesion affects intrarenal pressures.[33] However, it is a costly, invasive procedure that carries significant risks including hemorrhage, infection, arterial dissection, cholesterol embolization, allergic reaction, and nephrotoxicity, as well as the theoretical risks of radiation exposure. DSA is, therefore, usually reserved for confirmation of diagnosis and is typically performed in today's practice only before therapeutic interventional procedures. In select cases, carbon dioxide can be used as a contrast agent, thereby avoiding the risks associated with iodinated contrast at the expense of diminished contrast resolution.

Renal Vein Renin Sampling

Since RVH is caused by activation of the renin–angiotensin cascade, measurement of renin

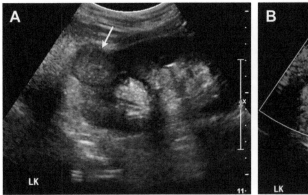
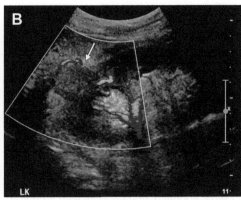

Fig. 5. Renal cell carcinoma. Gray scale (*A*) and power Doppler (*B*) sagittal images of the left kidney from a 63-year-old man with hypertension being evaluated to rule out renovascular hypertension (RVH) demonstrate an important incidental finding of an echogenic, vascular mass (*arrow*) at the upper pole consistent with a renal cell carcinoma.

released by an affected kidney is the most direct method of confirming the diagnosis of RVH. To measure renal vein renin levels, which will give functional information regarding the significance of a stenotic lesion, intravenous renal vein sampling must be performed. Typically the patient is premedicated with captopril, and plasma renin is measured via catheterization at the level of the upstream inferior vena cava (IVC) and in the renal veins. Pretreatment with captopril decreases renal perfusion pressures and thus enhances the effects of stenotic lesions.[34] The ratios of these measurements can be used to determine whether one or both kidneys are affected.[35] However, similar to intra-arterial DSA, this technique is invasive and exposes the patient to radiation, iodinated intravenous contrast, and other risks associated with catheterization.

Computed Tomography

Computed tomography (CT) angiography (CTA) provides fast, high-resolution anatomic assessment of the renal arteries. Beregi and colleagues[36] reported a sensitivity of 88% and a specificity of 98% for CTA in the detection of renal artery stenosis (RAS). CTA also has the advantage of visualizing secondary signs of renal artery stenosis, such as decreased cortical size or cortical thickness and delayed parenchymal contrast enhancement. In addition, CTA can evaluate for causes of renal artery stenosis such as extrinsic compression from a mass or congenital anomaly[37] and other causes of hypertension such as adrenal masses.[36,38] Despite these advantages, CTA requires the use of potentially nephrotoxic iodinated intravenous contrast and involves significant exposure to ionizing radiation.

Nuclear Medicine

The great advantage of using nuclear medicine to evaluate for RVH is that angiotensin-converting enzyme (ACE) inhibitor-enhanced renal scintigraphy, like renal vein sampling, demonstrates the functional significance of stenotic lesions. However, although ACE inhibitor renography has been reported in the literature to have extremely high sensitivity and specificity for the diagnosis of RVH, in the more unselected patient populations typically encountered in clinical practice, results are not nearly acceptable for screening purposes.[39] Additionally, scintigraphy provides no anatomic information. However, scintigraphy has a useful and often important complementary role with additional imaging techniques that provide anatomic information such as magnetic

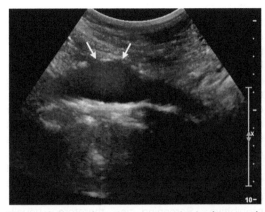

Fig. 6. Abdominal aortic aneurysm. Sagittal gray scale image of the abdominal aorta in a patient being evaluated for renal artery stenosis demonstrated an unsuspected infrarenal abdominal aortic aneurysm (*arrows*).

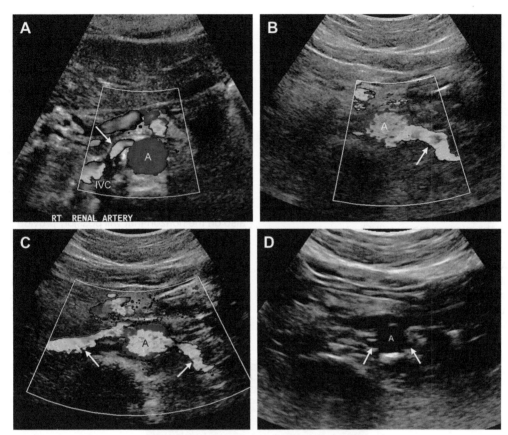

Fig. 7. Transverse midline images of the origins of the main renal arteries. (*A*) Color Doppler image of the origin of the right main renal artery (*arrow*). (*B*) Color Doppler image of the origin of the left MRA (*arrow*). (*C*) Color Doppler image of both main renal arteries (*arrows*). (*D*) Transverse gray scale image of the aorta depicting the origins of the main renal arteries (*arrows*). A, aorta; IVC, inferior vena cava.

resonance angiography (MRA).[40] Since scintigraphy depends on differential uptake or retention of radiotracer by the right and left kidneys, scintigraphy has a limited role in the evaluation of older patients who often have bilateral RAS. Although uptake and retention of radioisotope usually behave somewhat asymmetrically in patients with bilateral renal artery stenosis, scintigraphy actually has difficulty distinguishing between unilateral and bilateral disease.[41] Also, the examination essentially depends on renal function; thus renal insufficiency will also impair the sensitivity and specificity of the examination.[41]

Magnetic Resonance Imaging

MRA and Doppler ultrasound are currently the preferred noninvasive imaging modalities for evaluating patients with clinical concern for RVH. Although CT has higher spatial resolution than

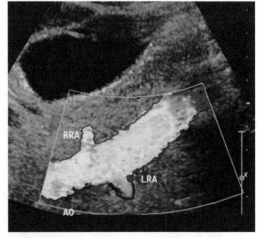

Fig. 8. Coronal or banana peel view of the aorta demonstrating the origins of the right and left main renal arteries. AO, aorta; LRA, left renal artery; RRA, right renal artery.

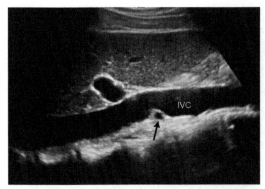

Fig. 9. Coronal gray scale image demonstrates the right renal artery in cross section (*arrow*) crossing under the inferior vena cava (IVC).

MRA, gadolinium-enhanced MRA reliably detects renal artery stenosis with a sensitivity of 97% and specificity of 93%, on par with CTA.[42] MRA does not use ionizing radiation but incurs higher costs than other modalities.[40] In the past, gadolinium contrast agents were thought to be safe in patients with renal impairment. It is now known that the administration of gadolinium to patients with renal failure can cause nephrogenic systemic fibrosis, a rare, potentially fatal disease.[43] Hence, gadolinium-enhanced MRA is now no longer considered a safe means of evaluating patients in renal failure with clinical suspicion of RVH. There are numerous investigational techniques undergoing evaluation directed toward performance of MRA without gadolinium, including time of flight, phase contrast, arterial spin labeling, and balanced steady-state free precession.[43–46] Quantitative measurements of renal perfusion with MRA are also on the horizon that will possibly provide functional and anatomic information in a single examination and could be performed with as little as 2 mL of gadolinium contrast.[47] Finally, magnetic resonance techniques in general are contraindicated for patients with most implantable medical devices. Some patients with claustrophobia cannot tolerate the smaller bore size of the

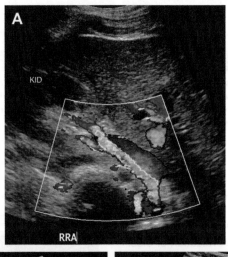

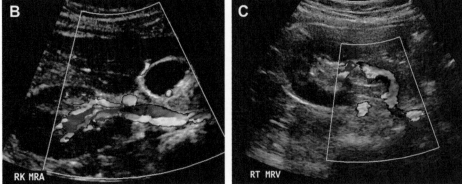

Fig. 10. (*A, B*) Parasagittal views through the renal hilum of the right kidney in two different patients demonstrate the entire length of the main renal artery (*red*). (*C*) This approach can also be used to evaluate the main renal vein (MRV) (*blue*). KID, right kidney.

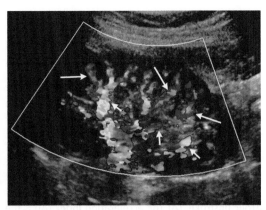

Fig. 11. Sagittal color Doppler image of the kidney demonstrates the segmental arteries (*short arrows*) within the echogenic renal sinus and the interlobar arteries (*long arrows*) lateral to the relatively hypoechoic renal pyramids.

magnetic resonance magnet compared with CT, and some patients are not able to breath hold adequately for the relatively longer acquisition times.

Doppler Ultrasound

Doppler ultrasound is noninvasive, relatively inexpensive, and uses no ionizing radiation. In many institutions, Doppler ultrasound is the preferred initial imaging modality in the work-up of suspected RVH, particularly in patients with renal dysfunction due to the risk of nephrogenic systemic fibrosis associated with gadolinium administration. In comparison to other imaging techniques, Doppler ultrasound provides physiologic assessment of stenotic lesions in addition to anatomic information, although the spatial resolution of Doppler ultrasound is inferior to DSA, CTA or MRA. As noted previously, documentation of the

hemodynamic significance of a stenosis in the renal artery is required to diagnose RVH, since patients with essential hypertension may have incidental, coexistent atherosclerotic stenotic lesions that do not trigger the renin-angiotensin-aldosterone cascade. Doppler ultrasound is primarily limited by operator dependence and technical failures because of nonvisualization of the renal arteries due to overlying bowel gas, aortic calcifications, and obesity, which limit penetration of the ultrasound beam, as well as inability of the patient to hold their breath. Intravenous ultrasound contrast (IVUC) agents are currently not approved for use in the United States, but IVUSC has agents have the potential to salvage otherwise nondiagnostic examinations. IVUSC agents such as lipid- or protein-stabilized microbubbles are intensely echogenic. They improve visualization of the renal arteries primarily by increasing backscatter.

Doppler Ultrasound Technique and Normal Findings

The kidneys are first examined with grayscale imaging. The maximum longitudinal renal length is measured. Renal cortical echogenicity and thickness are evaluated. The kidneys should be symmetric in length, cortical thickness, and echogenicity. Asymmetry of renal length (>1.5 cm), particularly if the smaller kidney has a thinner and more echogenic renal cortex, is suggestive of underlying renovascular pathology. Care should be taken to note any focal masses (**Fig. 5**), hydronephrosis, or nephrolithiasis. Grayscale imaging and color imaging of the aorta are also performed, with particular attention to search for plaque, thrombus, dissection (see **Fig. 3**), or aneurysm (**Fig. 6**), as these entities may involve the origins of the renal arteries. In addition, the presence of atherosclerosis in the aorta increases the pretest

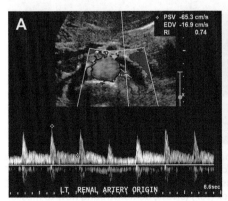
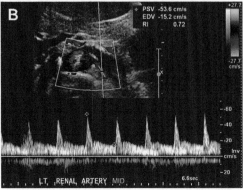

Fig. 12. Spectral Doppler tracings of the normal left main renal artery at the origin (*A*) and midpoint (*B*) demonstrate a sharp systolic upstroke and continuous forward diastolic flow.

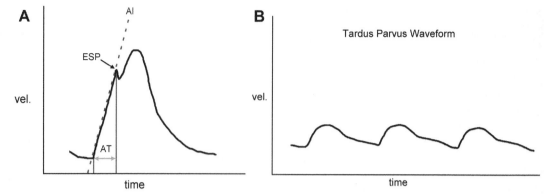

Fig. 13. Schematic diagrams demonstrating measures of systolic upstroke. (*A*) The acceleration index (AI) is the slope of the line between the onset of systole and the early systolic peak complex (ESP). The acceleration time (AT) is the length of time calculated by measuring along the baseline from the onset of systole to the ESP. Note that the ESP may not be observed in all patients (particularly the elderly). In many patients, the ESP corresponds to the peak systolic velocity (PSV), but in some patients the ESP may be lower than the peak systolic velocity. Acceleration time (AT) and index (AI) should be calculated in reference to the ESP even if it is lower than the second peak. However, the highest peak is used to calculate PSV. Increasing the frame rate will widen the Doppler tracing, making these calculations easier and more reproducible. (*B*) The tardus parvus waveform pattern is characterized by slow systolic upstroke as well as rounding and widening of a low velocity systolic peak.

probability of atherosclerotic stenosis at the origin of the renal arteries.

Doppler ultrasound is best performed with a 2 to 5 MHz curved array transducer, and the patient should fast for 8 to 12 hours before the examination to reduce attenuation of the ultrasound beam by air in overlying bowel. Harmonic imaging and spatial compounding techniques should be used if available. Color gain should be maximized until the image is degraded by color flash artifact from noise or patient motion, and then minimally reduced. Power Doppler ultrasound can increase sensitivity to slow flow and is less angle-dependent, but remains motion-dependent. In many cases, the use of color Doppler may facilitate identification of the renal arteries. On the other hand, the use of color Doppler decreases spatial resolution and frame rate, which may make the examination more difficult in patients who cannot adequately hold their breath. In these cases, using grayscale imaging alone without color Doppler may actually improve resolution and decrease motion artifact. The pulse repetition frequency (PRF) should be set high enough to prevent bleeding of color flow from adjacent veins or the main renal artery into the surrounding soft tissues and to reduce speckle artifact or noise from motion. However, the PRF should also be low enough such that the spectral

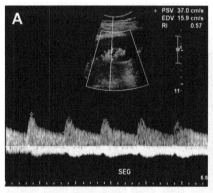
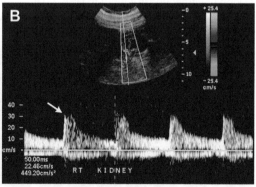

Fig. 14. Spectral Doppler tracings of normal intraparenchymal renal arteries. (*A*) A segmental artery demonstrating sharp systolic upstroke and continuous forward diastolic flow. There is no early systolic peak complex (ESP). The resistive index (RI) is 0.57. A normal RI is less than 0.70. Venous flow is noted below the baseline. (*B*) Spectral Doppler tracing in another patient with an early systolic peak complex (ESP) (*arrow*) demonstrating how to measure the AI and AT. The AT is 50 milliseconds. A normal AT is less than 70 milliseconds. The AI is 449 cm/s². Normal is greater than 300 cm/s².

Doppler waveform fills the entire scale and does not demonstrate aliasing at a site of stenosis. The Doppler sample volume should cover the entire width of the main renal artery, and the angle of insonation should be kept between 45° to 60° if possible. The angle is ideally kept constant on serial studies. Angles greater than 60° will artificially increase measured peak systolic velocities.

It is expected that several scanning planes and acoustic windows will be needed to visualize the entire length of the main renal artery. The origins of the main renal arteries are often best visualized using a transverse midline approach (**Fig. 7**). The main renal arteries usually arise anterolaterally just below the level of the left renal vein, which can be seen coursing across the midline, anterior to the aorta and under the superior mesenteric artery. Coronal images through the aorta, also known as the banana peel view, may sometimes be useful in displaying the origin of the renal arteries (**Fig. 8**). The right renal artery is the only vessel to course under the IVC and can be identified in cross section on coronal or sagittal images of the IVC (**Fig. 9**). An oblique parasagittal/coronal approach with the patient in a slight decubitus position, and angling through the renal hilum toward the aorta, can at times demonstrate the entire length of the main renal artery (**Fig. 10**).

Accessory renal arteries are usually not demonstrated on Doppler ultrasound due to their small size. However, if 2 vessels are identified exiting the renal hilum at the upper and lower poles, one should suspect the presence of multiple renal arteries or early branching of a single renal artery. Attempts should then be made to trace each vessel to the aorta.

The intraparenchymal renal arteries are best visualized using a translumbar lateral approach. The segmental arteries are found within the echogenic renal sinus. These in turn branch into the interlobar arteries, which course lateral to the pyramids (**Fig. 11**). The arcuate arteries run behind the pyramids parallel to the renal capsule.

Peak systolic velocity (PSV) is recorded in the main renal arteries at their origins, midpoint, and hilum (**Fig. 12**), as well as at any point along the length of the main renal artery that looks narrowed or demonstrates focal color aliasing. Ideally, the main renal arteries are sampled at 1 cm intervals along their entire length. The intraparenchymal interlobar or segmental arteries at the upper and lower poles are evaluated to obtain the acceleration index (AI), acceleration time (AT), and resistive index (RI). Three measurements at each pole should be obtained. The AI is the slope of the line, in meters per second squared, from the

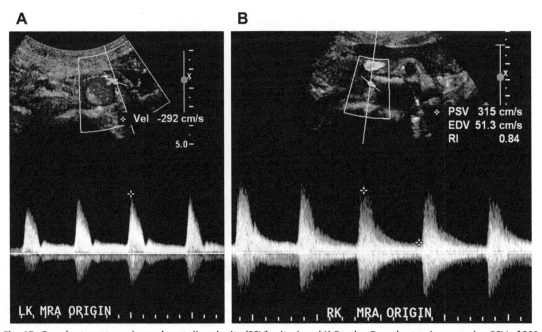

Fig. 15. Renal artery stenosis: peak systolic velocity (PSV) criterion. (*A*) Duplex Doppler tracing reveals a PSV of 292 cm/sec at the origin of the left MRA in an elderly patient with hypertension and renal failure. (*B*) In another patient with severe hypertension, PSV is 315 cm/s at the origin of the right main renal artery. In both patients PSV exceeds the threshold for the diagnosis of renal artery stenosis.

beginning of systole to the early systolic peak complex (ESP). The AT is the time, in milliseconds, from the beginning of systole to the early ESP (**Fig. 13A**). The authors refer to the ESP, because it does not necessarily correspond to the point of PSV, as some normal renal arteries demonstrate an early, lower systolic notch. Alternatively, the waveform may be subjectively evaluated for the presence of delayed systolic acceleration, a so-called tardus parvus waveform configuration which is characterized by a delayed systolic upstroke and rounded systolic peak of relatively low velocity (see **Fig. 13B**). In normal patients, the PSV in the main renal artery is less than 100 cm/s and decreases distally as one samples closer to the renal hilum. In the intraparenchymal renal arteries, the RI should measure less than 0.7, and the AT is less than 70 milliseconds (**Fig. 14**).

Diagnostic Ultrasound Criteria

Direct approach

A stenosis is generally considered hemodynamically significant at 50% to 60% diameter reduction, at which point, significant pressure gradients have been measured experimentally.[35] The ultrasound equivalent of this phenomenon is a focal increase in PSV to greater than 200 cm/s at the site of a stenosis (**Figs. 15** and **16**). On color Doppler, focal color aliasing, poststenotic turbulence, and post-stenotic dilatation may also be present. The threshold value of 200 cm/s has been shown to demonstrate a sensitivity of 85% and specificity of 92%.[48] Some authors advocate using a threshold PSV of 180 cm/s. Rarely, documentation of a focal increase in PSV in a distal hilar vessel may indicate a branch stenosis (**Fig. 17**). A ratio calculated by

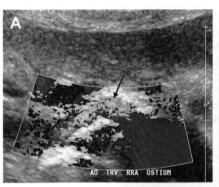
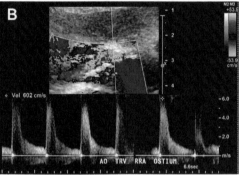
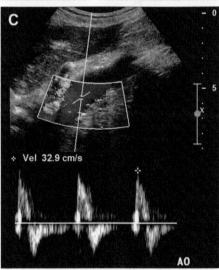

Fig. 16. Renal artery stenosis. (*A*) Color Doppler image of a patient with refractory hypertension reveals focal color aliasing at the origin of the right main renal artery (*arrow*), narrowing of the main renal artery, and a color soft tissue bruit in the surrounding soft tissues due to perivascular tissue vibration due to increased velocity of blood flowing through the stenosis. (*B*) Peak systolic velocity (PSV) in the right main renal artery is 690 cm/s in comparison to a PSV 36 of cm/s in the aorta (*C*). The renal to aortic PSV ratio (RAR) is nearly 20. Although the RAR dramatically exceeds the threshold value of 3.5 for the diagnosis of RAS, the RAR may not be highly accurate in diagnosis (ie, loses specificity) when the aortic PSV is this low.

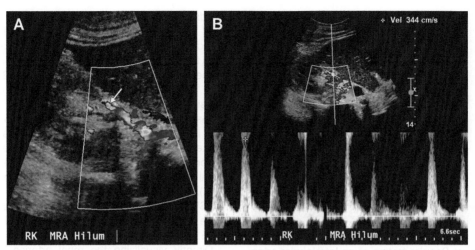

Fig. 17. Stenosis of a branch vessel. (*A*) Note narrowing and focal color aliasing (*arrow*) of a branch vessel in the right renal hilum. (*B*) Spectral tracing reveals a PSV of 344 cm/s in comparison to 80 cm/s in other hilar arteries (not shown). Findings are consistent with stenosis in an arterial branch to the upper pole of the right kidney. Stenoses in branch vessels are unusual but can occasionally be seen in patients with atherosclerosis.

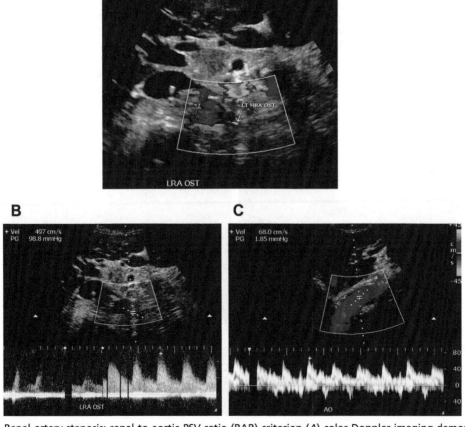

Fig. 18. Renal artery stenosis: renal to aortic PSV ratio (RAR) criterion (*A*) color Doppler imaging demonstrates marked narrowing at the origin if the left renal artery in a 64-year-old woman with hypertension and renal failure. (*B*) PSV is 497 cm/s in comparison to a PSV of 68 cm/s in the aorta (*C*). The RAR is 7.3. Findings are consistent with high-grade renal artery stenosis.

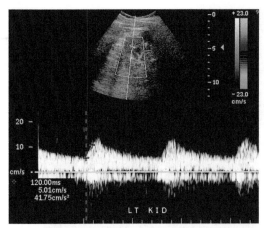

Fig. 19. Renal artery stenosis: tardus parvus (TP) waveform pulse Doppler tracing of an interlobular artery from the left kidney demonstrates a slow systolic upstroke (AT = 120 m/s; normal AT = 70 m/s) as well as rounding and flattening of a low-velocity (12 cm/s) systolic peak. Although not seen in all patients with renal artery stenosis, a TP waveform is strongly suggestive of a more proximal stenosis. Elderly patients with long-standing hypertension, atherosclerosis, or diabetes often have stiff vessels with poor compliance, which blunts the development of the TP waveform distal to a stenosis. Conversely, preadminstration of 25 mg of captopril will accentuate the TP waveform phenomenon. (*Reprinted from* Moukaddam H, Pollak J, Scoutt LM. Imaging renal artery stenosis. US Clin 2007;2:66; with permission.)

dividing the PSV in the main renal artery by the PSV in the aorta, called the renal-to-aortic peak systolic velocity ratio (RAR), is thought to compensate for variations in cardiac output. This is used at some centers, and an RAR greater than 3.5 (see **Fig. 16; Fig. 18**) has been shown to have up to a sensitivity of 91% and similar specificity.[49] Decreasing the threshold cutoff from 3.5 to 2.5 or 3.0 increases sensitivity and is advocated at some institutions. Alternatively, Li and colleagues[50] propose using the ratio of the PSV in the main renal artery to the PSV in the renal-interlobar ratio (RIR). In his study, an RIR greater than 5 and a PSV less than 15 cm/s in the interlobar arteries were shown to have a sensitivity and specificity of 91% and 87%, respectively.[50]

Directly visualizing the renal arteries can be technically challenging due to dyspnea, obesity, overlying bowel gas, and shadowing from aortic calcifications, and in most institutions despite careful optimization of technique, the main renal arteries are not completely visualized in up to 30% of patients.[51] Cardiac arrhythmias and poor angles of insonation can further complicate accurate estimation of PSV. Accessory renal arteries occur in 15% to 24% of patients,[52–54] but are rarely seen on ultrasound due to their small size. Fortunately, in the rare event (<1%), that a stenosis is present in an accessory renal artery, it is unlikely to cause RVH.[55,56] Similarly, it is extremely difficult to visualize stenosis occurring at branch points in the hilar vessels in most patients (see **Fig. 17**).

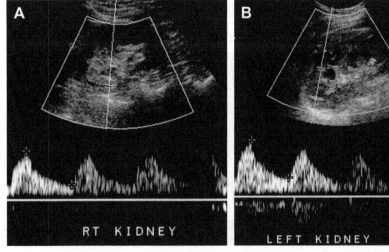

Fig. 20. Aortic stenosis. (*A, B*) Bilateral mild tardus parvus (TP) waveforms are noted bilaterally in the intraparenchymal vessels in a patient with severe aortic stenosis. The TP waveform is not specific for renal artery stenosis, but merely indicates the presence of a proximal stenosis. Bilateral TP intrarenal waveforms can be seen in patients with bilateral renal artery stenosis, narrowing of the aorta, or aortic stenosis.

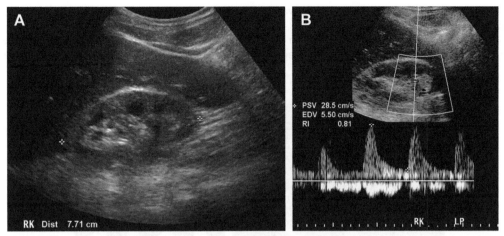

Fig. 21. (A) Gray scale image demonstrates a small (7.7 cm) right kidney with an echogenic renal cortex. (B) On Doppler interrogation, the RI is 0.81. Despite the fact that this hypertensive 62-year-old woman had an angiographically demonstrated renal artery stenosis greater than 80% of the right main renal artery, revascularization might not improve either blood pressure or renal function due to pre-existing end organ damage suggested by the elevation of the intraparenchymal RI.

Indirect approach

Instead of directly visualizing a stenosis in the main renal artery, one may look for an indirect effect of the stenosis on the waveform of the distal intraparenchymal renal arteries. A significant stenosis will theoretically cause a downstream delay in systolic acceleration. This delay can be recognized as a prolongation of the AT or as a decrease in the slope from the onset of systole to the early peak systolic complex, or acceleration index (AI). A tardus parvus waveform also indicates a more proximal stenosis (**Fig. 19**). This delay in systolic acceleration is not observed in the main renal artery but distally in the intraparechymal renal arteries. As a Doppler tracing of the intraparenchymal renal arteries can be successfully obtained in virtually all patients who can hold their breath, indirect Doppler evaluation for RVH by searching for a tardus parvus waveform or other measure of delay in systolic acceleration such as prolonged AT or slow AI in the intraparenchymal renal arteries is significantly easier to perform than the direct approach that requires visualization of the entire length of the main renal artery. Stavros and colleagues[57] reported that using an AT greater than 70 milliseconds showed a sensitivity and specificity of 78% and 94%, respectively, for a hemodynamically significant renal artery stenosis greater than 60%. In his series, an AI less than 3 m/s^2 had a sensitivity and specificity of 89% and 83%, respectively,[57] In addition, visual inspection of the waveform itself for tardus parvus (rounding and flattening of the systolic peak) has also been touted as a method of choice. Stavros and colleagues[57] concluded that visual

inspection surpassed numerical methods, with sensitivity of 95% and specificity of 97%.

However, delay in systolic acceleration does not always occur distal to a stenosis, since any process that increases peripheral vascular resistance and decreases compliance of the renovascular tree can block this phenomenon.[55] Hence, the tardus parvus waveform may not develop in older patients or patients with diabetes, atherosclerosis, or longstanding hypertension due to increased peripheral vascular resistance as well as increased stiffness

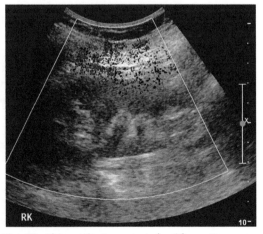

Fig. 22. This patient presented with acute, severe right flank pain following stent placement in the right renal artery. Sagittal color Doppler image reveals no blood flow in the right kidney, consistent with occlusion of the stent/renal artery, in this case secondary to dissection of the renal artery during the procedure.

and decreased compliance of the vessel walls. Unfortunately, these processes are also risk factors for ARVD. The attenuation of the delay in systolic acceleration can potentially be mitigated by preadministration of 25 mg captopril 1 hour before the Doppler ultrasound examination, which will accentuate the development of the tardus parvus phenomenon in patients with renal artery

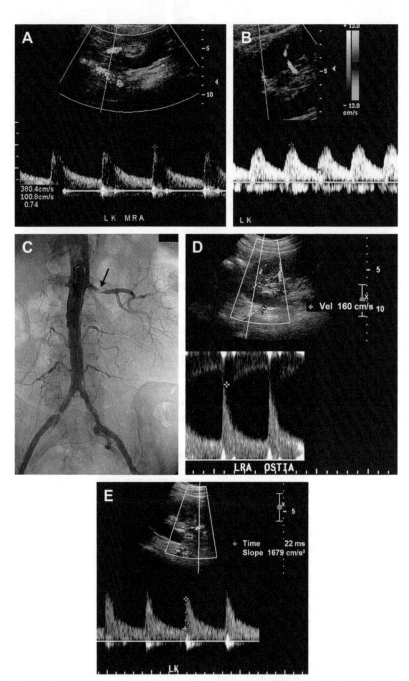

Fig. 23. Successful stent placement in a 68-year-old woman with severe hypertension and occluded right renal artery. Although peak systolic velocity (PSV) likely demonstrates compensatory increase in a renal artery contralateral to an occluded renal artery, PSV in the left renal artery is 380 cm/s (*A*), consistent with a high-grade stenosis. (*B*) Distal tardus parvus (TP) waveforms were also seen. (*C*) Angiogram demonstrates a tight stenosis in the proximal third of the left main renal artery (*arrow*). (*D*) Following stent placement, PSV in the main renal artery drops to 160 cm/s and a sharp systolic upstroke (AT = 22 cm/s) is now seen in the intraparenchymal vessels (*E*).

stenosis.[58] In addition, a decrease in the rate of systolic acceleration is not a specific finding for renal artery stenosis. Any proximal extrarenal stenosis such as aortic coarctation (see **Fig. 4**), severe aortic stenosis (**Fig. 20**), and William-Beuren syndrome (in children) (see **Fig. 2**) can all provoke a decrease in the rate of systolic acceleration, mimicking renal artery stenosis, although the tardus parvus waveform will be noted bilaterally in such cases. In addition, it has been postulated that reduced force of left ventricular contraction as may occur in patients with left ventricular dysfunction, left ventricular or aortic aneurysms and perhaps even afterload reducing cardiac medications, may also decrease the rate of systolic acceleration distally. Collateral blood flow in patients with renal artery occlusions often demonstrates decreased rate of systolic acclereration, mimicking renal artery stenosis. Furthermore, measurement of the AT, AI, and waveform analysis have also been reported to have significant inter- and intraobserver variability.[59–61]

PREOPERATIVE ASSESSMENT

Given the recent controversy regarding the lack of improvement in outcome of patients with RVH who undergo revascularization in comparison to medical therapy alone, more attention is being focused on improving patient selection, with the idea that only carefully selected patient populations will likely benefit from revascularization.[62] On the other hand, for patients with more severe disease such as bilateral RAS, renal dysfunction, recurrent pulmonary edema, or unstable angina, the impetus to intervene is greater.[62] Furthermore, patients with higher blood pressure preoperatively have the greatest decreases in systolic blood pressure after stenting.[63] Imaging can be helpful to select patients as well. For example, patients with bilateral RAS and normal kidney parenchymal thickness are more likely to respond to revascularization with durable drop in blood pressure or improvement in renal function.[63,64] Conversely, if the kidney is small with a thin, echogenic renal cortex, end-organ damage has likely already occurred, and revascularization may be fruitless (**Fig. 21**).

It is controversial whether the RI can help predict patient response to revascularization. It has been postulated that increased RI implies irreversible end-organ damage, and in 2001 Radermacher and colleagues[65] reported that patients with a RI greater than 0.8 in the intraparenchymal vessels were less likely to demonstrate improvement in blood pressure control or renal function following revascularization procedures (see **Fig. 21**). However, other authors suggest that while an elevated RI may correlate with poor blood pressure response, it does not predict the likelihood of achieving improvement in renal function.[66] Another group reported that patients with or without elevated RI achieved similar improvements in blood pressure and renal function after revascularization at 6-month follow-up, although patients without elevated RI were more likely to be able to reduce the number of antihypertensive medications and that renal function was more likely to continue to improve over the long term.[67]

POSTOPERATIVE ASSESSMENT

Doppler ultrasound has been successfully used to assess stent patency after revascularization. In contrast, MRA and CTA have difficulty depicting the residual lumen following stent placement due to artifact from the wall of the stent. Immediately postrevascularization, Doppler ultrasound may be helpful by demonstrating patency of the main and intraparenchymal renal arteries to exclude thrombosis or embolus in patients presenting with acute flank pain, hematuria, or decreased renal function following surgery or more commonly

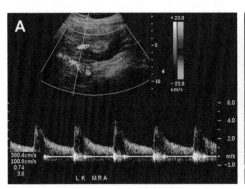 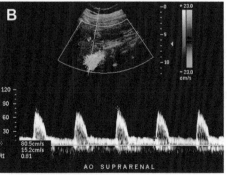

Fig. 24. In stent restenosis—same patient as in **Fig. 23**. 18 months after stent placement, blood pressure has become elevated again. (A) Peak systolic velocity (PSV) is 380 cm/s within the stent in comparison to 80 cm/s in the aorta (B) with renal to aortic PSV ratio (RAR) of 4.75. Findings are consistent with in-stent restenosis.

following percutaneous stenting or balloon angioplasty (**Fig. 22**). In the case of acute thrombus or embolus following revascularization, immediate accurate diagnosis is critical so that blood flow may be reestablished as quickly as possible to prevent irreversible renal infarction. If revascularization is technically successful, PSV in the main renal artery should decrease. Delayed systolic acceleration should normalize, and the systolic upstroke should become sharp (**Fig. 23**). In-stent restenosis occurs in up to 15% of patients and can be clinically occult.[68,69] The Doppler ultrasound criteria for restenosis are still evolving, and reports vary from laboratory to laboratory, possibly related to stent type and diameter, with PSV thresholds ranging from 144 to 226 cm/s and RAR from 2.7 to 3.5 (**Fig. 24**).[70,71] There is also a theoretical concern that stents decrease vessel wall compliance, leading to false-positive elevation of peak systolic velocities. Hence, diagnostic thresholds are likely to be higher for stented renal arteries in comparison to the native renal artery. Restenosis status post surgical bypass can also occur. However, despite this concern and general experience, at least 1 laboratory has reported that sensitivity and specificity for restenosis using criteria for native arteries (PSV >180 cm/s) were comparable to using customized laboratory specific criteria.[72]

FUTURE TRENDS

Although used widely in other countries including Canada and Europe, intravenous ultrasound contrast agents are currently investigational in the United States and have not yet been approved by the US Food and Drug Administration. These agents are typically microbubbles containing perfluorocarbon gas stabilized by an outer lipid or protein coating. Since gas is intensely reflective of the ultrasound beam, intravenous ultrasound contrast agents increase the returning ultrasound signal, primarily by increasing backscatter; they thus have the potential to dramatically increase the sensitivity of an ultrasound vascular examination. By highlighting the blood vessel lumen, these agents have the potential to salvage technically limited examinations[73,74] due to depth, body habitus, and inability to hold one's breath. However, the administration intravenous ultrasound contrast agents can introduce color blooming artifact andnoise; they may also artificially increase measured PSV.[75] Despite these concerns, administration of intravenous ultrasound contrast agents does not seem to interfere with sensitivity or specificity of Doppler ultrasound examination for RVH.[76,77]

One of the newest developments in ultrasound is elastography, which measures tissue deformation under strain. This investigational technique has already found numerous potential applications, from imaging thyroid nodules to breast masses. In renovascular ultrasound application, measurement of perivascular tissue vibrations with elastogrpahy techniques has been proposed as a mechanism of diagnosing stenosis of the main renal artery indirectly without the need to visualize the arterial lumen itself.[78]

SUMMARY

Doppler ultrasound is an inexpensive, noninvasive screening method for the diagnosis of renovascular hypertension. It provides both anatomic and functional information in a single study, aiding clinicians in preoperative and postoperative assessment for potential intervention, without the risks of radiation, nephrotoxicity, or nephrogenic systemic fibrosis. The main limitation of Doppler ultrasound is technical failure to visualize the entire length of the main renal arteries. In the future, the use of intravenous ultrasound contrast agents and elastography holds promise to reduce the rate of technical failure.

REFERENCES

1. Egan BM, Zhao Y, Axon RN. US trends in prevalence, awareness, treatment, and control of hypertension, 1998-2008. JAMA 2010;303:2043–50.
2. Garovic VD, Textor SC. Renovascular hypertension and ischemic nephropathy. Circulation 2005;112: 1362–74.
3. Goldblatt H, Lynch J, Hanzal RF, et al. Studies on experimental hypertension: I. The production of persistent elevation of systolic blood pressure by means of renal ischemia. J Exp Med 1934;59: 347–79.
4. Textor SC, Wilcox CS. Renal artery stenosis: a common treatable cause of renal failure? Annu Rev Med 2001;52:421–42.
5. Cheung CM, Hegarty J, Kalra PA. Dilemmas in the management of renal artery stenosis. Br Med Bull 2005;73-74:35–55.
6. Hansen KJ, Edwards MS, Craven TE, et al. Prevalance of renovascular disease in the elderly: a population-based study. J Vasc Surg 2002;36:443–51.
7. Zierler RE, Bergelin RO, Davidson RC, et al. A prospective study of disease progression in patients with atherosclerotic renal artery stenosis. Am J Hypertens 1996;9:1055–61.
8. Caps MT, Perissinotto C, Zierler RE, et al. Prospective study of atherosclerotic disease progression in the renal artery. Circulation 1998;98:2866–72.

9. Caps MT, Zierler RE, Polissar NL, et al. Risk of atrophy in kidneys with atherosclerotic renal artery stenosis. Kidney Int 1998;53:734–42.

10. Tollefson DF, Ernst CB. Natural history of atherosclerotic renal artery stenosis associated with aortic disease. J Vasc Surg 1991;14:327–31.

11. Schreiber MJ, Pohl MA, Novick AC. The natural history of atherosclerotic and fibrous renal artery disease. Urol Clin North Am 1984;11:383–92.

12. Zeller T. Renal artery stenosis: epidemiology, clinical manifestation, and percutaneous endovascular therapy. J Interv Cardiol 2005;18:497–506.

13. Ives NJ, Wheatley K, Stowe RL, et al. Continuing uncertainty about the value of percutaneous revascularization in atherosclerotic renovascular disease: a meta-analysis of randomized trials. Nephrol Dial Transplant 2003;18:298–304.

14. ASTRAL Investigators, Wheatley K, Ives N, et al. Revascularization versus medical therapy for renal artery stenosis. N Engl J Med 2009;361:1953–62.

15. Neymark E, LaBerge JM, Hirose R, et al. Arteriographic detection of renovascular disease in potential renal donors: incidence and effect on donor surgery. Radiology 2000;214:755–60.

16. Rabelink TJ, Wijewickrama DC, de Koning EJ. Peritubular endothelium: the Achilles heel of the kidney? Kidney Int 2007;72:926–30.

17. Shanley PF. The pathology of chronic renal ischemia. Semin Nephrol 1996;16:21–32.

18. Margoles HR, Trerotola SC. Fibromuscular dysplasia of the brachial artery causing hemodialysis access dysfunction. J Vasc Interv Radiol 2009;20:1087–9.

19. Rice RD, Armstrong PJ. Brachial artery fibromuscular dysplasia. Ann Vasc Surg 2010;24:255.

20. Najafi AH, Wang Z, Kent KM. Fibromuscular dysplasia of ostial left main coronary artery depicted by intravascular ultrasound. Cardiovasc Revasc Med 2009;10:277–9.

21. Yano T, Kasahara Y, Tanabe N, et al. Juvenile pulmonary hypertension associated with fibromuscular dysplasia. Intern Med 2010;49:2487–92.

22. Kincaid OW, Davis GD, Hallermann FJ, et al. Fibromuscular dysplasia of the renal arteries arteriographic features, classification, and observations on natural history of the disease. Am J Roentgenol Radium Ther Nucl Med 1968;104:271–82.

23. Trinquart L, Mounier-Vehier C, Sapoval M, et al. Efficacy of revascularization for renal artery stenosis caused by fibromuscular dysplasia. A systematic review and meta-analysis. Hypertension 2010;56: 525–32.

24. Barrier P, Julien A, Canevet G, et al. Technical and clinical results after percutaneous angioplasty in nonmedial fibromuscular dysplasia: outcome after endovascular management of unifocal renal artery stenoses in 30 patients. Cardiovasc Intervent Radiol 2010;33:270–7.

25. Jain S, Kumari S, Ganguly NK, et al. Current status of Takayasu arteritis in India. Int J Cardiol 1996;54:S111–6.

26. Sharma BK, Sagar S, Chugh KS, et al. Spectrum of renovascular hypertension in the young in north India: a hospital based study on occurrence and clinical features. Angiology 1985;36:370–8.

27. Kumar A, Dubey D, Bansal P, et al. Surgical and radiological management of renovascular hypertension in a developing country. J Urol 2003;170:727–30.

28. Rose C, Wessel A, Pankau R, et al. Anomalies of the abdominal aorta in Williams-Beuren syndrome—another cause of arterial hypertension. Eur J Pediatr 2001;160:655–8.

29. Pankau R, Partsch CJ, Winter M, et al. Incidence and spectrum of renal abnormalities in Williams-Beuren syndrome. Am J Med Genet 1996;63:301–4.

30. Ingelfinger JR, Newburger JW. Spectrum of renal anomalies in patients with Williams syndrome. J Pediatr 1991;119:771–3.

31. Daghero F, Bueno N, Peirone A, et al. Coarctation of the abdominal aorta: an uncommon cause of arterial hypertension and stroke. Circ Cardiovasc Imaging 2008;1:e4–6.

32. Delis KT, Gloviczki P. Middle aortic syndrome: from presentation to contemporary open surgical and endovascular treatment. Perspect Vasc Surg Endovasc Ther 2005;17:187–203.

33. Cam A, Chhatriwalla AK, Kapadia S. Limitations of angiography for the assessment of renal artery stenosis and treatment implications. Catheter Cardiovasc Interv 2010;75:38–42.

34. Lyons DF, Streck WF, Kem DC, et al. Captopril stimulation of differential renins in renovascular hypertension. Hypertension 1983;5:615–22.

35. Simon G. What is critical renal artery stenosis? Implications for treatment. Am J Hypertens 2000;13: 1189–93.

36. Beregi JP, Elkohen M, Deklunder G, et al. Helical CT angiography compared with arteriography in the detection of renal artery stenosis. Am J Roentgenol 1996;167:495–501.

37. Gaebel G, Hinterseher I, Saeger HD, et al. Compression of the left renal artery and celiac trunk by diaphragmatic crura. J Vasc Surg 2009;50:910–4.

38. Wittenberg G, Kenn W, Tschammler A, et al. Spiral CT angiography of renal arteries: comparison with angiography. Eur Radiol 1999;9:546–51.

39. Huot SJ, Hansson JH, Dey H, et al. Utility of captopril renal scans for detecting renal artery stenosis. Arch Intern Med 2002;162:1981–4.

40. Bolduc JP, Oliva VL, Therasse E, et al. Diagnosis and treatment of renovascular hypertension: a cost–benefit analysis. Am J Roentgenol 2005;184:931–7.

41. Mann SJ, Pickering TG, Sos TA, et al. Captopril renography in the diagnosis of renal artery stenosis: accuracy and limitations. Am J Med 1991;90: 30–40.

42. Tan KT, van Beek EJ, Brown PW, et al. Magnetic resonance angiography for the diagnosis of renal artery stenosis: a meta-analysis. Clin Radiol 2002; 57:617–24.

43. Cowper SE, Su LD, Bhawan J, et al. Nephrogenic fibrosing dermopathy. Am J Dermatopathol 2002;23: 383–93.

44. Roditi G, Maki JH, Oliveira G, et al. Renovascular imaging in the NSF era. J Magn Reson Imaging 2009;30:1323–34.

45. Glockner JF, Takahashi N, Kawashima A, et al. Noncontrast renal artery MRA using an inflow inversion recovery steady state free precession technique (Inhance): comparison with 3D contrast-enhanced MRA. J Magn Reson Imaging 2010;31:1411–8.

46. Xu JL, Shi DP, Li YL, et al. Nonenhanced MR angiography of renal artery using inflow-sensitive inversion recovery pulse sequence: a prospective comparison with enhanced CT angiography. Eur J Radiol 2010. [Epub ahead of print].

47. Lee VS, Rusinek H, Johnson G, et al. MR renography with low-dose gadopentetate dimeglumine: feasibility. Radiology 2001;221:371–9.

48. Williams GJ, Macaskill P, Chan SF, et al. Comparative accuracy of renal duplex sonographic parameters in the diagnosis of renal artery stenosis: paired and unpaired analysis. Am J Roentgenol 2007;188:798–811.

49. Soares GM, Murphy TP, Singha MS, et al. Renal artery duplex ultrasonography as a screening and surveillance tool to detect renal artery stenosis a comparison with current reference standard imaging. J Ultrasound Med 2006;25:293–8.

50. Li JC, Wang L, Jiang YX. Evaluatiton of renal artery stenosis with velocity parameters of Doppler sonography. J Ultrasound Med 2006;25:735–42.

51. Desberg AL, Pauschter DM, Lammert GK, et al. Renal artery stenosis: evaluation with color Doppler flow imaging. Radiology 1990;177:749–53.

52. Helenon O, El Rody F, Correas JM, et al. Color Doppler US of renovascular disease in native kidneys. Radiographics 1995;15:833–54.

53. Berland LL, Koslin DB, Routh WD, et al. Renal artery stenosis: prospective evaluation of diagnosis with color duplex US compared with angiography. Radiology 1990;174:421–3.

54. Geyer JR, Poutasse EF. Incidence of multiple renal arteries on aortography. JAMA 1962;182:120–5.

55. Bude RO, Forauer AR, Caoili EM, et al. Is it necessary to study accessory arteries when screening the renal arteries for renovascular hypertension? Radiology 2003;226:411–6.

56. Gupta A, Tello R. Accessory renal arteries are not related to hypertension risk: a review of MR angiography data. Am J Roentgenol 2004;182:1521–4.

57. Stavros AT, Parker SH, Yakes WF, et al. Segmental stenosis of the renal artery: pattern recognition of tardus and parvus abnormalities with duplex sonography. Radiology 1992;184:487–92.

58. Rene PC, Oliva VL, Bui BT, et al. Renal artery stenosis: evaluation of Doppler US after inhibition of angiotension-converting enzyme with captopril. Radiology 1995;196:675–9.

59. Keogan MT, Kliewer MA, Hertzberg BS, et al. Renal resistive indices: variability in Doppler US measurement in a healthy population. Radiology 1996;199: 165–9.

60. Kliewer MA, Hertzberg BS, Keogan MT, et al. Early systole in the healthy kidney: variability of Doppler US waveform parameters. Radiology 1997;205:109–13.

61. Gottlieb RH, Snitzer EL, Hartley DF, et al. Interobserver and intraobserver variation in determining intrarenal parameters by Doppler sonography. Am J Roentgenol 1997;168:627–31.

62. Henry M, Benjelloun A, Henry I, et al. Renal angioplasty and stenting: is it still indicated after ASTRAL and STAR studies? J Cardiovasc Surg 2010;51: 701–20.

63. White CJ, Olin JW. Diagnosis and management of atherosclerotic renal artery stenosis improving patient selection and outcomes. Nat Clin Pract Cardiovasc Med 2009;6:176–90.

64. Zeller T, Frank U, Muller C, et al. Predictors of improved renal function after percutaneous stent-supported angioplasty of severe atherosclerotic ostial renal artery stenosis. Circulation 2003;108:2244–9.

65. Radermacher J, Chavan A, Bleck J, et al. Use of Doppler ultrasonography to predict the outcome of therapy for renal-artery stenosis. N Engl J Med 2001;344:410–7.

66. Garcia-Criado A, Gilabert R, Nicolau C, et al. Value of Doppler sonography for predicting clinical outcome after renal artery revascularization in atherosclerotic renal artery stenosis. J Ultrasound Med 2005;24: 1641–7.

67. Zeller T, Muller C, Frank U, et al. Stent angioplasty of severe atherosclerotic ostial renal artery stenosis in patients with diabetes mellitus and nephrosclerosis. Catheter Cardiovasc Interv 2003;58:510–5.

68. Isles CG, Robertson S, Hill D. Management of renovascular disease: a review of renal artery stenting in ten studies. QJM 1999;92:159–67.

69. Oertle M, Do DD, Baumgartner I, et al. Discrepancy of clinical and angiographic results in the follow-up of percutaneous transluminal renal angioplasty (PTRA). Vasa 1998;27:154–7.

70. Bakker J, Beutler JJ, Elgersma OEH, et al. Duplex ultrasonography in assessing restenosis of renal artery stents. Cardiovasc Intervent Radiol 1999;22: 475–80.

71. Napoli V, Pinto S, Bargellini I, et al. Duplex ultrasonographic study of the renal arteries before and after renal artery stenting. Eur Radiol 2002;12: 796–803.

72. Fleming SH, Davis RP, Craven TE, et al. Accuracy of duplex sonography scans after renal artery stenting. J Vasc Surg 2010;52:953–7.

73. Melany ML, Grant EG, Duerinckx AJ, et al. Ability of a phase shift US contrast agent to improve imaging of the main renal arteries. Radiology 1997;205:147–52.

74. Claudon M, Plouin PF, Baxter GM, et al. Renal arteries in patients at risk of renal artery stenosis: multicenter evaluation of the echo-enhancer SH U 508A at color and spectral Doppler US. Radiology 2000;214:739–46.

75. Forsberg F, Liu JB, Burns PN, et al. Artifacts in ultrasonic contrast agent studies. J Ultrasound Med 1994;13:357–65.

76. Teixeria OU, Bortolotto LA, Silva HB, et al. The contrast-enhanced Doppler ultrasound with perfluorocarbon exposed sonicated albumin does not improve the diagnosis of renal artery stenosis compared with angiography. J Negat Results Biomed 2004;3:3.

77. Blebea J, Zickler R, Volteas N, et al. Duplex imaging of the renal arteries with contrast enhancement. Vasc Endovascular Surg 2003;37: 429–36.

78. Sikdar S, Vaidya S, Dighe M, et al. Doppler vibrometry: assessment of arterial stenosis by using perivascular tissue vibrations without lumen visualization. J Vasc Interv Radiol 2009;20:1157–63.

Vascular Complications of Liver Transplants: Evaluation with Duplex Doppler Ultrasound

Stephanie A. Reid, MD[a], Leslie M. Scoutt, MD[b], Ulrike M. Hamper, MD, MBA[c],*

KEYWORDS

- Liver transplantation • Vascular complications
- Doppler duplex ultrasound • Sonographic evaluation

Since the first successful cadaveric liver transplantation performed by Thomas Starzl in 1967, liver transplantation has evolved into the treatment of choice for patients with end-stage liver disease and early hepatic malignancies.[1] Advances in surgical techniques and improvement in post-transplant medical care have led to continued improvement in morbidity and mortality. However, despite the advances, postoperative complications still arise and cause significant morbidity and mortality in graft recipients. The most dreaded complications are vascular in nature, the most severe of which is hepatic arterial thrombosis, which is associated with the worst outcome.

Ultrasound is the initial imaging modality of choice in the postoperative liver transplant because of its portability, noninvasiveness, and its ability to detect complications. This article focuses on the sonographic evaluation of vascular complications following liver transplantation. To recognize complications, it is important to have a basic understanding of surgical techniques and knowledge of the spectrum of normal appearances, which is also reviewed.

LIVER TRANSPLANTATION TODAY

Liver transplantation is the treatment of choice for a variety of end-stage liver disorders. In adults, the most common indications for transplant are cirrhosis caused by hepatitis C virus, alcoholic liver disease, or cryptoenic/unknown causes followed by cholestatic liver diseases such as primary sclerosing cholangitis and primary biliary cirrhosis.[2] Metabolic or genetic disorders such as Wilson disease and hemochromatosis, acute fulminant hepatic failure, cirrhosis caused by hepatitis B virus, Budd-Chiari syndrome, and primary hepatic malignancies are less common indications.[2]

The authors have nothing to disclose.
[a] Russell H. Morgan Department of Radiology and Radiological Science, The Johns Hopkins University School of Medicine, Nelson B106, 600 North Wolfe Street, Baltimore, MD 21287, USA
[b] Department of Diagnostic Radiology, Yale University School of Medicine, 333 Cedar Street, PO Box 208042, New Haven, CT 06520-8042, USA
[c] Ultrasound Section, Russell H. Morgan Department of Radiology and Radiological Science, The Johns Hopkins University School of Medicine, Nelson B106, 600 North Wolfe Street, Baltimore, MD 21287, USA
* Corresponding author.
E-mail address: umhamper@jhu.edu

doi:10.1016/j.cult.2011.07.003
1556-858X/11/$ – see front matter © 2011 Elsevier Inc. All rights reserved.

Prioritization for liver allocation in the United States uses the Model of End-Stage Liver Disease (MELD) score, which is an objective measurement based on serum creatinine, serum total bilirubin, and international normalized ratio (INR) of prothrombin time.[3] The MELD score has been shown to accurately predict liver disease severity and mortality, and thus serves as an effective tool for liver allocation.[4] Liver transplantation has also been proved to be an effective treatment of small, unresectable hepatocellular carcinomas (HCC) in patients with cirrhosis.[5] A single HCC measuring less than or equal to 5 cm, or up to 3 HCC tumor nodules measuring 3 cm or less in diameter, known as the Milan criteria, generally serve as the guidelines for defining transplant eligibility in patients with HCC.[5]

Based on Organ Procurement and Transplantation Network (OPTN) data, 6320 liver transplants were performed in 2009. However, based on OPTN data as of January 21, 2011, there are currently 16,765 patients on the waiting list for a liver transplant. The discrepancy between the limited number of available donor organs and the large number of patients awaiting liver transplants has prompted efforts to expand the donor pool. This expansion has included the development of partial liver grafts using split liver cadaveric and living donor transplants. The initial success in reduced-size liver transplants in pediatric patients led to the use and subsequent evolution of surgical techniques for partial liver grafts in adult recipients.[6] Living donor transplantation has a risk to the donor and remains limited in the United States, with only 219 performed in 2009 according to OPTN, compared with 6101 cadaveric.[7] However, living donor liver transplants provide most grafts in Asian countries because of a limited supply of cadaveric liver donors.[8]

SURGICAL TECHNIQUES
Cadaveric Whole-liver Orthotopic Liver Transplantation

Liver transplantation is orthotopic, meaning the donor liver is placed in the anatomic location of the removed native liver. Liver transplantation requires 4 surgical anastomoses: 1 biliary and 3 vascular (venous, portal, and arterial), each of which is reviewed in detail.

Biliary Anastomosis

The biliary anastomosis is usually an end-to-end anastomosis between the recipient common bile duct and the donor common bile duct, referred to as a choledochocholedochostomy.[9] In patients with an inadequate common bile duct (small, short, or diseased) a choledochojejunostomy is performed. Choledochojejunostomy is less preferable because of the lack of preservation of the sphincter of Oddi, associated bacterial overgrowth related to enteric reflux, and subsequent increased risk of infection.[10] A cholecystectomy is routinely performed following transplantation.[9]

Venous Anastomosis

The venous anastomosis is variable. The conventional technique is an end-to-end anastomosis of the donor and recipient inferior vena cava (IVC). The recipient IVC segment is removed with the liver and the donor IVC is anastomosed with the suprahepatic and infrahepatic IVC remnants of the recipient (Fig. 1).[11] A second method, the piggyback technique, preserves the recipient IVC with a single anastomosis performed between a common cuff formed from the recipient hepatic veins and the donor suprahepatic IVC in an end-to-side anastomosis (Fig. 2). The donor infrahepatic IVC is oversewn.[12] A modified piggyback technique uses a side-to-side cavocaval anastomosis. A longitudinal incision is made in the posterior wall of the donor IVC and the anterior wall of the recipient wall, which are anastomosed in a side-to-side fashion. The suprahepatic and infrahepatic donor IVC are oversewn.[13]

Portal Venous Anastomosis

The portal venous anastomosis is typically an end-to-end portoportal anastomosis (Fig. 3).[11] In the event of recipient portal vein (PV) thrombosis (PVT), a jump interposition graft between the donor PV and the recipient superior mesenteric vein is performed, usually using a donor iliac vein.[14]

Arterial Anastomosis

A branch patch technique is often used for the arterial anastomosis, with the branch patch of the recipient formed at the origin of the gastroduodenal artery from the common hepatic artery anastomosed to the branch patch of the donor, usually formed at the branch point of the common hepatic and splenic arteries versus a Carrel patch of celiac axis.[15] Variant hepatic artery anatomy necessitates additional back-table preparation and more complicated arterial reconstructions.[15–17] In the event of recipient hepatic artery or celiac axis high-grade stenosis, an aortohepatic interposition graft using donor iliac artery may be used. This method involves anastomosis of the graft to the recipient hepatic artery and to the aorta in an end-to-side anastomosis.[17]

Important considerations for arterial anastomoses and vascular anastomoses in general include near-equal donor and recipient vessel diameter and lack of surplus vessel length to

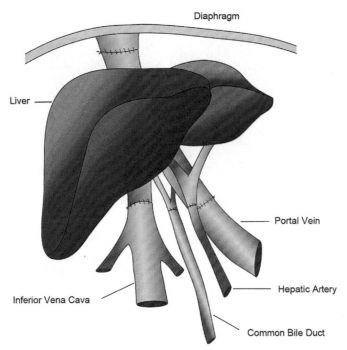

Fig. 1. Surgical anastomoses. The conventional end-to-end IVC anastomosis. The portal vein (PV), hepatic artery, and common bile duct anastomoses are also shown.

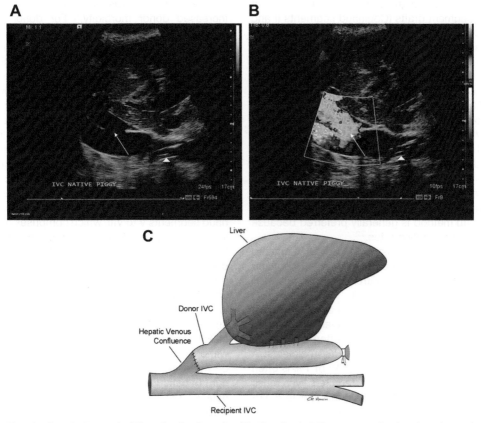

Fig. 2. Piggyback IVC. Grayscale (*A*) and color Doppler (*B*) piggyback IVC anastomosis, showing the end-to-side anastomosis (*arrow*). IVC filter is present inferior to the anastomosis (*arrowhead*). (*C*) Piggyback anastomosis.

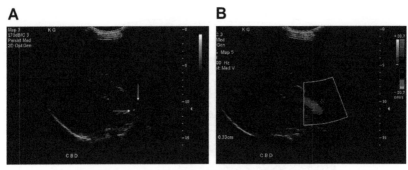

Fig. 3. PV anastomosis. Grayscale (*A*) and color Doppler (*B*) images of an end-to-end portal venous anastomosis, with echogenic foci along the periphery of the PV wall representing surgical material (*arrows*).

decrease the risk for subsequent vascular complications.

Reduced-size Liver Transplantation, Split Liver, and Living Donor Liver Transplantation

The unique segmental nature of liver anatomy and its extensive regenerative potential allow for a variety of partial hepatic grafts.[18,19] Reduced-size liver transplantation (RLT) was first developed in pediatric patients, primarily to fill the large need for adequate-sized grafts in this population.[20] Left lateral segment grafts (Couinaud segments II and III) and left hepatic lobe grafts (Couinaud segments II, III, and IV) are most commonly used in the pediatric patient.[20] Initially, the remainder of the partial donor graft was discarded. However, Pichlmayr and colleagues[21] in 1988 reported the first attempt at split liver transplantation, using a single donor liver for 2 grafts. An extended right graft (segments I, IV–VIII) was transplanted into an adult and a left lateral graft (segments II, III) was transplanted into a child. Both ex vivo splitting (following explantation, performed on the bench) and in situ splitting (before explantation, while still in the heart beating donor) techniques have been developed; however, the in situ method is generally preferred because of lower complication rates.[22]

Living donor liver transplantation (LDLT) marked another expansion in the potential donor pool and was first successfully introduced in pediatric patients in 1989.[23] In 1993, LDLT was then expanded to adult patients, with a left lobe graft transplanted in an adult.[24] However, it was soon discovered that left lobe grafts often provide an insufficient hepatic volume for adult recipients. A graft/recipient weight ratio (GRWR) of 1% is often used as an estimate of the required liver mass needed for a hepatic transplant in order to maintain sufficient metabolic function in the recipient.[25] Posttransplant liver dysfunction is more commonly seen with GRWR of less than 1%.[25] If donor body size is less than that of the recipient, the left lobe is usually inadequate and places the recipient at risk for small-for-size graft syndrome.[8] Small-for-size grafts show enhanced parenchymal cell injury, prolonged cholestasis, and delayed synthetic function, which, overall, can lead to lower graft survival.[25]

As a result, LDLT using right lobe grafts was introduced in adults in 1996.[26] Although improving recipient survival, right lobe transplantations impart an increased risk to the donor because of reduced volume of residual liver, which results in increased donor morbidity.[7] For donor safety, donation is only recommended when the estimated remnant liver volume is greater than 30%.[27] LDLT remains rare in the United States, accounting for less than 5% of the overall number of liver transplantations performed. However, LDLT accounts for greater than 90% of the total number of liver transplantations in Asia because of high need and lack of supply of cadaveric livers.[8]

LDLT and split liver transplantation are technically challenging, with smaller caliber ducts and vessels requiring complicated anastomoses and reconstructions. The most common graft currently used in adult LDLT is the right hepatic lobe, Couinaud segments V to VIII, which comprises approximately 60% of whole liver volume.[9] The preferred biliary anastomosis is duct to duct, with graft bile duct anastomosed to recipient common hepatic duct; however, roux-en-Y hepaticojejunostomy can also be performed.[28] The arterial anastomosis is typically between the donor right hepatic artery and the recipient common hepatic artery.[9] Because the donor right hepatic graft is procured without the IVC, venous anastomosis is typically between donor right hepatic vein and recipient right hepatic vein with a caval extension or, alternately, from the donor right hepatic vein to a common trunk formed by the recipient's hepatic vein orifices.[9] Continuing advances in surgical techniques have led to improvements in biliary and hepatic venous complications, which were initially high in LDLT.[28,29] To improve venous drainage of the anterior sector of the graft and prevent complications from venous congestion, techniques of an extended right lobe graft to include the middle hepatic vein trunk versus reconstruction of anterior sector veins and use of venous interposition grafts are often used.[29]

Postoperative Ultrasound, Normal and Abnormal Findings

Doppler duplex sonography is an important tool in the postoperative liver transplant for early diagnosis of postoperative complications. Many transplant centers use protocols for routine liver duplex ultrasound screening in the postoperative period to aid in early detection of complications before clinical signs or symptoms arise. Early detection with early intervention can potentially decrease morbidity and mortality associated with transplant complications.[30]

Sonographic evaluation of the postoperative liver transplant consists of grayscale examination of the liver and right upper quadrant with grayscale, color Doppler, and duplex Doppler evaluation of the hepatic arteries, PVs, hepatic veins, and IVC. When interpreting early postoperative studies, a clear understanding of the spectrum of normal appearances is important in order to recognize true complications.

Hepatic Artery, Normal Appearance

Pulsed Doppler waveform of a normal hepatic artery shows a low-resistance waveform with continuous forward diastolic flow with a sharp systolic upstroke (**Fig. 4**).[31] Normal parameters include a systolic acceleration time (SAT; time from end-diastole to the first systolic peak) of

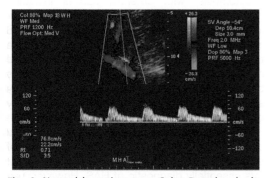

Fig. 4. Normal hepatic artery. Color Doppler duplex image of the main hepatic artery showing a normal hepatic arterial waveform, with a sharp systolic upstroke and a normal resistive index of 0.71 (normal range 0.55–0.80).

less than 80 milliseconds and a resistive index (RI; the difference of the peak systolic velocity [PSV] and peak diastolic velocity [PDV] divided by the peak systolic velocity, RI = PSV−PDV/PSV) between 0.55 and 0.80.[32]

In the early postoperative period, particularly in the first 72 hours, hepatic artery resistive indices may be temporarily increased without clinical significance or adverse prognosis (**Fig. 5**).[33] Early increased RIs have been associated with older donor age (>50 years old) and extended preservation.[33] Without clinical suspicion of hepatic artery complications, increased RIs with documented arterial flow can generally be followed with sequential ultrasounds.[31,33] Additional imaging with noninvasive computed tomographic angiography (CTA)/magnetic resonance angiography (MRA) or invasive conventional angiography should be performed if no arterial flow is shown on duplex ultrasound, RI increase persists (particularly in the absence of diastolic flow and diminished systolic flow), or if there is clinical suspicion of a hepatic arterial complication.[31,33]

Hepatic Artery Complications

Posttransplantation hepatic artery complications include hepatic artery thrombosis (HAT), stenosis, and pseudoaneurysms.

HAT

HAT is the most common vascular complication and also the most severe, with high associated morbidity and mortality. The reported incidence of HAT ranges from approximately 3% to 12% in adult transplant recipients, with more recently reported data in the lower end of this range.[30,34–37] In an analysis of 15 transplant centers with a total of 7185 orthotopic liver transplantations performed, Strange and colleagues[34] reported that the average incidence of HAT was approximately 5%. However, the significance lies in the associated graft failure and mortality, with a mean retransplantation rate of 53% (with a range of 25%–83%) and average mortality of 31% (with a range of 9%–55%). A meta-analysis of early HAT, which reviewed 71 studies and 21,822 transplants, revealed similar findings. Overall early HAT rate was 4.4% with a mortality of 33.3% and retransplantation rate of 53.1%.

HAT can be subdivided into early and delayed phases based on the time of occurrence following surgery. There is some variability in the literature of the definition of early thrombosis, but it is generally considered early if it occurs within 30 days of transplantation.[38] Numerous risk factors for HAT have been reported, but many were found to be

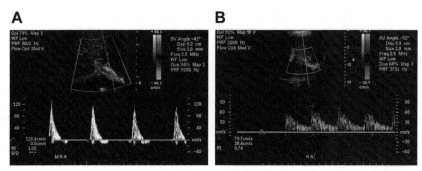

Fig. 5. Initial postoperative findings. (*A*) Color Doppler duplex image of the main hepatic artery on postoperative day #1 showing abnormal high-resistance arterial waveform with lack of forward diastolic flow, mild early reversal of diastolic flow, and a resistive index of 1.0. (*B*) Follow-up color Doppler duplex image of the main hepatic artery 5 days later showing a normal hepatic arterial waveform with normal resistive index of 0.74. Increased RI can be seen temporarily in the early postoperative period.

discordant in a recent meta-analysis of early HAT.[39] Some concordant risk factors for HAT that have been reported include pediatric patients, retransplantation, CMV serology status mismatch between donor and recipient, low recipient weight, low-volume transplant centers, arterial variants/reconstructions, and prolonged operation time.[38]

Unlike in a normal liver, in which the biliary tree has a dual blood supply by the PV and hepatic artery, the posttransplant biliary tree is solely dependent on the hepatic artery for its blood supply. With interruption of the blood supply caused by thrombosis, biliary ischemia can result. The clinical presentation of HAT can range from fulminant hepatic failure/necrosis to delayed biliary leaks and recurrent bacteremia to less severe allograft dysfunction.[30,35,40] On imaging studies, the sequelae of HAT can be visualized, including infarctions, bilomas, and abscesses.

Doppler ultrasound of early HAT classically shows no identifiable arterial blood flow within the main hepatic artery or intrahepatic arteries (**Fig. 6**).[41] To prevent a false-positive interpretation, care must be taken to distinguish decreased arterial flow, which can be seen in severe hepatic edema, high-grade hepatic artery stenosis, increased central venous pressures, or systemic hypotension, from the true absence of flow.[42] Arterial collaterals can develop in the porta hepatitis in patients with HAT, more commonly in the delayed form, and the collateral flow can be confused with main hepatic artery flow and cause a false-negative interpretation.[31] However, in this situation, intra-arterial waveforms are typically abnormal, showing a tardus-parvus appearance with delayed systolic acceleration times (>0.8 milliseconds) and low resistive indices (<0.5) (**Fig. 7**).[41]

Investigators Nolten and Sproat[42] describe a pattern of hepatic arterial flow on serial duplex

ultrasounds seen before thrombosis, labeled as the syndrome of impending thrombosis. Typically in a span of 3 to 10 days, successive examinations show a progressive decline in diastolic flow followed by a decrease in systolic flow and, ultimately, complete loss of arterial signal.[42]

If HAT is suspected on ultrasound, it may be confirmed with CTA/MRA versus conventional angiogram. Revascularization with surgical thrombectomy or, less often, endovascular thrombolysis, can be attempted if the HAT is diagnosed promptly.[34,43] However, retransplantation is required in the event of graft failure.[30,34] If sufficient collateralization of flow is present and graft function is preserved, patients can be managed nonoperatively with observation.[30]

Hepatic Artery Stenosis

Hepatic artery stenosis (HAS) has an incidence of approximately 4% to 11%.[30,35,44] The most common site of stenosis is at or near the arterial anastomosis, with potential causes including clamp injury, disruption of the vasa vasora, or intimal trauma.[41] The clinical presentation of HAS is variable, ranging from mild hepatic dysfunction to graft failure secondary to biliary ischemia and necrosis.[45] If left untreated, hepatic artery stenosis can progress to complete occlusion caused by slow flow, emphasizing the importance of early detection.[41]

Color Doppler and duplex imaging of HAS show aliasing and turbulence just distal to the site of stenosis, with an increased PSV greater than 2 m/s essentially diagnostic of HAS. However, use of this criteria alone limits sensitivity for HAS detection, because the hepatic artery may not be visualized in its entirety because of obscuration by bowel gas. In these situations when the site of

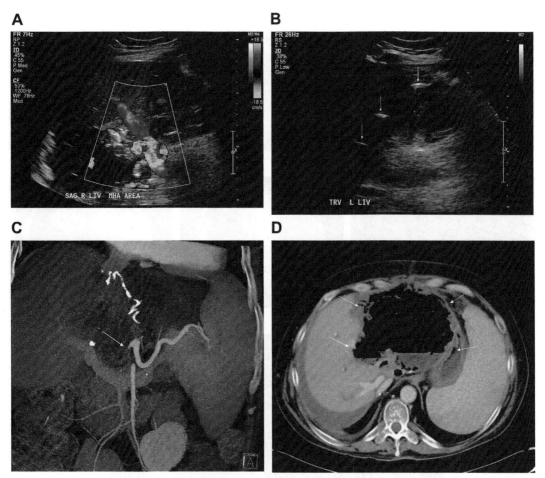

Fig. 6. HAT. (*A*) Color Doppler image with low scale showing no color flow in the region of the main hepatic artery. (*B*) Grayscale image of the left hepatic lobe showing poor definition of the left hepatic lobe with bright linear echoes, suspicious for gas (*arrows*). (*C*) Coronal volume-rendered image from contrast-enhanced CT showing thrombosis of the proximal main hepatic artery (*arrow*). (*D*) Axial contrast-enhanced CT image showing large collection of gas within the left hepatic lobe, compatible with infarction and abscess, sequelae of HAT (*arrows*).

stenosis is not directly visualized, intrahepatic artery waveforms can indirectly suggest more proximal stenosis. Intrahepatic arteries typically show a tardus-parvus waveform with prolonged systolic acceleration time (>0.8 milliseconds) and low resistive indices (<0.5) (**Fig. 8**).[41] However, as mentioned previously, similar intrahepatic waveforms can be seen in the setting of chronic HAT with collateralization.[41]

It is important to evaluate both the main hepatic artery as well as the intrahepatic arteries, because stenoses can occur anywhere along the arterial course.[45] In addition, in the event of variant arterial anatomy, awareness of the surgical reconstruction technique is critical to fully evaluate the hepatic arterial system.[45] If tardus-parvus waveforms are visualized within the main hepatic artery, the celiac axis should be evaluated for stenosis. Most

commonly, celiac artery stenosis is secondary to atheromatous disease, but median arcuate ligament syndrome should be considered in the younger patient.[10]

Suspected HAS is often confirmed with CTA/MRA or conventional angiography. Treatment with minimally invasive percutaneous transluminal angioplasty with or without stent placement is generally preferred; however, surgical correction is also a treatment option and may be necessary in the immediate postoperative period.[44,46]

Hepatic Artery Pseudoaneurysm

Hepatic artery pseudoaneurysm (PA) is an uncommon vascular complication following transplant, occurring in 0.6% to 2%.[35,47,48] Although uncommon, there is a high associated mortality

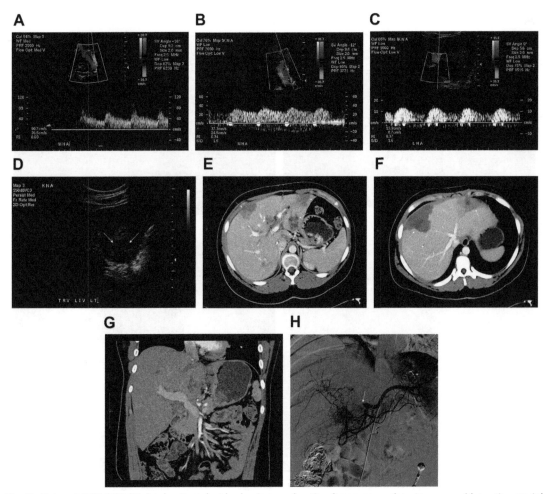

Fig. 7. Delayed HAT. (*A*) Initial color Doppler duplex image shortly after surgery showing normal hepatic arterial waveform and normal resistive index (0.60) in the main hepatic artery. Four months later, color Doppler duplex images of the main hepatic artery (*B*) and left hepatic artery (*C*) show tardus-parvus waveforms with increased diastolic flow and abnormal resistive indices of 0.34 and 0.37, respectively. (*D*) Grayscale image of the liver shows irregular hypoechoic focus within the periphery of the left hepatic lobe, suspicious for infarct (*arrows*). (*E*)Axial contrast-enhanced CT image at this same level also shows this irregular hypoechoic focus in the left hepatic lobe, as well as additional peripheral hypodense foci, compatible with infarcts (*arrows*). (*F*) Additional axial CT image more superiorly shows classic wedge-shaped areas of infarction (*arrows*). (*G*) Coronal contrast-enhanced volume-rendered image showing thrombosis of the main hepatic artery (*arrow*). (*H*) Arteriogram performed 2 months later shows thrombosis of the main hepatic artery (*arrow*) with extensive small collaterals supplying the liver.

because of the consequences of rupture.[47] The most common cause of extrahepatic PA is local infection, with the most common site of occurrence at the arterial anastomosis. Patients with a roux-en-Y hepaticojejunostomy anastomosis are at greater risk for PA because of increased bacterial colonization at the porta hepatitis.[47] In addition, surgical technical difficulties at the arterial anastomosis, pancreatitis, and systemic infection are also associated with increased risk of extrahepatic PA.[47] Risk factors for development of intrahepatic artery pseudoaneurysms include prior percutaneous interventions such as liver

biopsy, percutaneous transhepatic cholangiography, or transhepatic drainage catheters.[47]

Clinically, pseudoaneurysms often go undiagnosed until patients present with life-threatening hemorrhage following rupture.[47,49] Intrahepatic PA rupture may lead to arterioportal or arteriobiliary fistula.[10] Early diagnosis of this unsuspected complication on ultrasound can be critical to patient survival.[49]

Grayscale imaging of a nonthrombosed hepatic artery PA shows a rounded anechoic structure along the course of the hepatic artery. Color and spectral Doppler analysis classically show flow

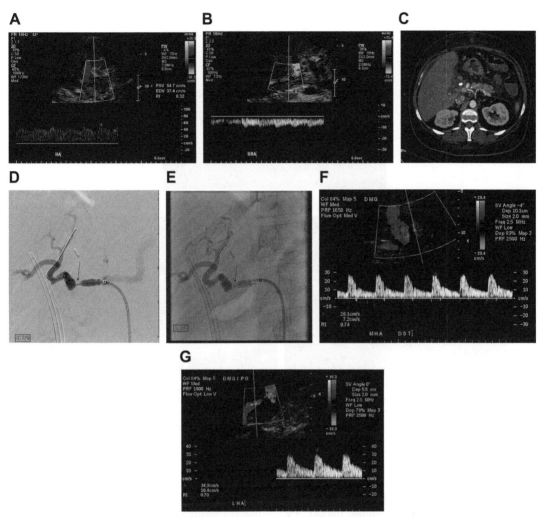

Fig. 8. HAS. Color Doppler duplex images of the main hepatic artery (*A*) and right hepatic artery (*B*) showing tardus-parvus waveforms with increased diastolic flow and abnormal resistive indices (0.32 in the main hepatic artery). (*C*) Axial arterial phase contrast-enhanced CT image shows high-grade focal stenosis in the main hepatic artery (*arrow*) with poststenotic dilatation. (*D*) Arteriogram before balloon angioplasty also showing the high-grade focal stenosis in the main hepatic artery (*arrow*). (*E*) Second arteriogram image following balloon angioplasty showing improvement in the degree of stenosis, with mild residual stenosis (*arrow*). Color Doppler duplex image of the main hepatic artery (*F*) and left hepatic artery (*G*) following angioplasty showing a return to normal hepatic arterial waveforms with normal resistive indices (0.74 and 0.70, respectively).

within the lumen in a to-and-fro pattern (yin-yang appearance) (**Fig. 9**) and disorganized arterial waveform in the neck. If an anechoic structure is encountered on a postoperative transplant ultrasound, color Doppler and spectral Doppler analysis should be performed to differentiate a vascular complication from a fluid collection.[49] With intraluminal thrombosis, a PA may be difficult to distinguish from postoperative hematoma.[47]

Extrahepatic pseudoaneurysms are typically treated surgically with resection and revascularization. Elective repair is preferred because of poor outcomes associated with emergent revascularization after rupture.[47] Percutaneous embolization can be performed as a temporary measure with the understanding that potential interruption of hepatic arterial blood supply may lead to graft failure and the need for retransplantation.[47] Intrahepatic pseudoaneurysms are typically treated with embolization.[48]

PV, Normal Appearance

Spectral Doppler analysis of a normal PV shows continuous forward laminar flow toward the liver (hepatopetal) with mild undulations secondary to

A

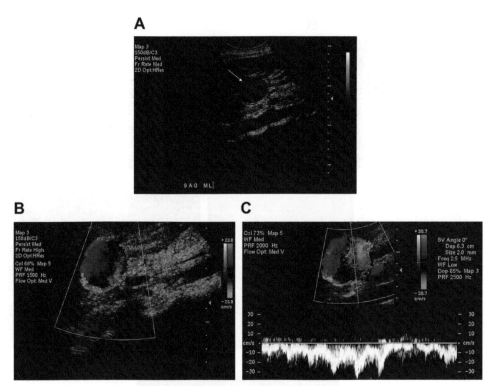

Fig. 9. Hepatic artery PA. (*A*) In a nontransplant liver, grayscale image near the porta hepatis shows a large, rounded anechoic structure (*arrow*). (*B*) Color Doppler image reveals classic to-and-fro flow (yin-yang appearance) in the anechoic structure, compatible with pseudoaneurysm. (*C*) Color Doppler duplex images show disorganized arterial flow. Pseudoaneurysm in a liver transplant patient would have an identical appearance.

respirations (**Fig. 10**).[10] However, in up to 43% of patients in the early postoperative period, PV flow is helical, meaning spiral flow, which is overall hepatopetal.[50] With helical flow, color Doppler shows regular alternating red and blue bands.

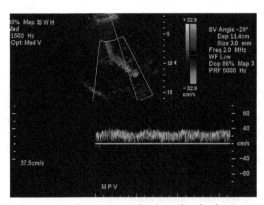

Fig. 10. Normal main PV. Color Doppler duplex image of the main PV showing normal hepatopetal flow and a monophasic waveform with mild undulations, reflecting mild respiratory variations.

Spectral Doppler tracings vary depending on placement of the cursor, with hepatopetal flow, hepatofugal flow, or both shown, depending on where sampled. This helical pattern of flow typically occurs with a size discrepancy between donor and recipient PVs and usually resolves within weeks. However, persistent helical flow can be seen with PV stenosis (PVS) or a significant size discrepancy.[50] It is important to distinguish between helical flow and true bidirectional flow, flow above and below the baseline, which can be seen in portal venous hypertension and thrombosis.

Normal PV velocities are typically less than 50 to 58 cm/s/s.[51,52] However, transient increases in PV velocities can be seen in the immediate postoperative period, likely because of compressibility caused by postoperative inflammation or fluid collections (**Fig. 11**).[51,53]

PV complications

PV complications include stenosis and thrombosis. PV aneurysm formation is an extremely rare occurrence in the liver transplant patient. Overall, PV complications are less common than

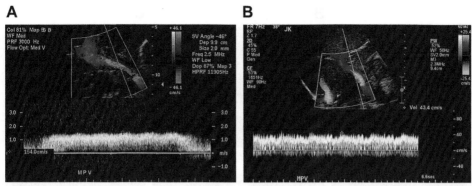

Fig. 11. Initial postoperative findings. (*A*) Color Doppler duplex image of the main PV on postoperative day #1 showing apparent luminal narrowing with associated high velocity in the main PV, 154 cm/s/s. (*B*) Follow-up imaging performed 3 months later revealed normal PV velocity (43 cm/s/s) and no evidence of narrowing. Temporary increased velocities can be seen in the immediate postoperative period. The initial findings were likely caused by postoperative edema.

hepatic arterial complications in cadaveric whole-liver transplantations, with incidences ranging from 1% to 2.7%.[35,54] However, the complication rate is reportedly higher in LDLT.[55]

PVT

Early clinical presentation of PVT may include acute hepatic failure or edema. Late presentations include signs and symptoms of severe portal hypertension, including ascites and esophageal variceal bleeding.[54] Risk factors for PVT include modified PV anastomoses, such as end to end to the confluence of the superior mesenteric vein (SMV) and splenic vein (SV) or venous interposition graft, and alterations to the PV wall, such as with prior thrombosis and recanalization.[54] Additional risk factors in LDLT for PVT include smaller-sized grafts, use of cryopreserved vein grafts, and PVT at time of transplant.[56]

Grayscale imaging of PVT typically shows intra-luminal echogenic thrombus within the PV.[10] However, grayscale images may appear near normal if the thrombus is acute and anechoic or

hypoechoic (**Fig. 12**A).[10] Color and duplex Doppler imaging shows no or decreased intraluminal flow, depending on the degree of thrombosis (see **Fig. 12**B). Bidirectional flow may be seen before thrombosis (**Fig. 13**).[54]

Treatment of PVT depends on the degree of occlusion, time of thrombosis, and clinical circumstances. Acute PVT treatment can include surgical thrombectomy or interposition graft placement; however, retransplantation may be required in the event of graft failure.[54] Local antithrombolysis therapy or transjugular intrahepatic portosystemic shunt (TIPS) procedures are also treatment options.[54]

PVS

PVS may be asymptomatic if the stenosis is mild; however, higher degrees of stenosis (>80%) are more often symptomatic, presenting with signs and symptoms of portal hypertension.[54]

Parameters for detecting PVS are variable in the literature, with most criteria described being sensitive, but not specific for its identification. In general,

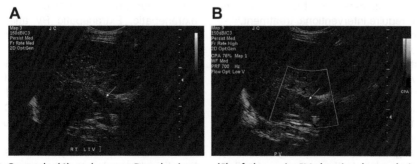

Fig. 12. PVT. Grayscale (*A*) and power Doppler images (*B*) of the main PV showing hypoechoic intraluminal thrombus within the main PV with lack of flow on power Doppler, compatible with PVT (*arrow*).

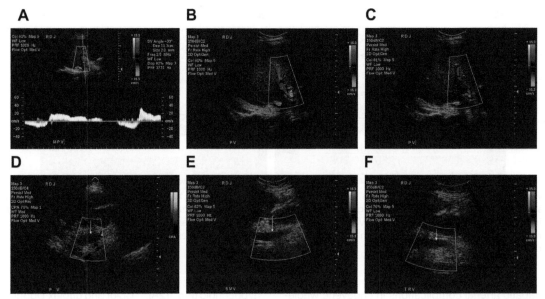

Fig. 13. Bidirectional PV flow in the setting of proximal PV, SMV, and splenic vein thrombosis. (*A*) Color Doppler duplex image of the main PV showing flow above and below the baseline, compatible with bidirectional PV flow. (*B, C*) Color Doppler images of the main PV showing alternating hepatopetal (*red*) and hepatofugal (*blue*) flow in the main PV, respectively. (*D*) Power Doppler image of the PV confluence and color Doppler images of the SMV (*E*) and splenic vein (*F*) showing intraluminal hypoechoic thrombus and absence of internal flow (*arrow*). (*From* Friedewald SM, Molmenti EP, DeJong MB, et al. Vascular and nonvascular complications of liver transplants: sonographic evaluation and correlation with other imaging modalities and findings at surgery and pathology. Ultrasound Quarterly 2003;19:80; with permission.)

grayscale imaging of PVS typically shows a focal area of luminal narrowing, with color and spectral Doppler showing aliasing and turbulence distal to the stenosis (**Fig. 14**).[46] Indirect signs of PVS can include visualizing stigmata of portal hypertension, including splenomegaly and varices.[55]

Huang and colleagues[57] describe 2 Doppler ultrasound parameters for detecting PVS in adult LDLT, a PV stenotic ratio greater than 50% (prestenotic caliber—anastomotic site caliber/prestenotic caliber) and a velocity ratio greater than 3:1 between the anastomotic site and the preanastomotic site. The investigators also found that an anastomotic site diameter less than 5 mm was more likely to require interventional treatment.[57]

Chong and colleagues[51] reported that using the parameters of a peak velocity greater than 125 cm/s or an anastomotic/preanastomotic velocity ratio of 3:1 achieves a specificity of 95% or greater for detection of PV anastomotic stenosis. However, Mullan and colleagues[58] report using a PV velocity measurement of greater than 80 cm/s with a change in velocity greater than 60 cm/s/s across the stenotic segment. The discrepancy in velocity parameters may relate to the presence of collaterals, decreasing velocity measurements.[58]

Treatment is dependent on the clinical situation and can include conservative management versus angioplasty with or without stent placement.[46,54,59] Surgical resection of the anastomotic segment with reconstruction is also a consideration.[60]

PV aneurysms are a rare occurrence, with only a few case reports described in patients after liver transplantation.[61,62] In patients not receiving transplants, PV aneurysms have been attributed to portal hypertension or congenital causes.[63] However, the cause of PV aneurysms in patients receiving transplants is less clear.

PV aneurysms are classified as intrahepatic or extrahepatic. Extrahepatic PV aneurysms have been defined as fusiform or saccular dilatation of the main PV, with luminal diameter greater than 19 to 21 mm (**Fig. 15**).[61,63] Intrahepatic aneurysms have been defined by Koc and colleagues[63] as greater than 9 mm in diameter and significantly larger than adjacent PV segments. Color Doppler duplex shows internal turbulent venous flow within the PV aneurysm.

Clinically, smaller aneurysms are usually asymptomatic, whereas larger aneurysms are more often symptomatic and associated with complications

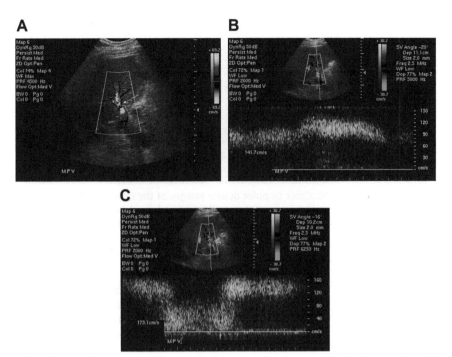

Fig. 14. PVS. (*A*) Color Doppler image of the main PV showing focal area of luminal narrowing with associated aliasing (*arrow*). (*B, C*) color Doppler duplex images reveal significantly increased PV velocities, 142 cm/s/s and 173 cm/s/s, suggesting PVS.

including thrombosis, portal hypertension, or biliary tract obstruction caused by mass effect.[63] Treatment depends on the size and clinical situation, and can include observation versus surgical resection.[63]

IVC and Hepatic Veins, Normal

Normal flow in the hepatic veins is toward the IVC (hepatofugal) with spectral tracings showing triphasic waveforms, reflecting nearby cardiac cycle variations (**Fig. 16A**).[10] IVC flow is also triphasic, often more pronounced than in the hepatic veins, reflecting the closer proximity to the heart (see **Fig 16B**). In the early postoperative period, loss of the normal triphasic waveform may be seen without clinical significance.[51] However, if triphasic venous waveforms are initially seen and become monophasic on follow-up examinations, acute rejection, IVC thrombosis, or IVC compression should be considered.[64]

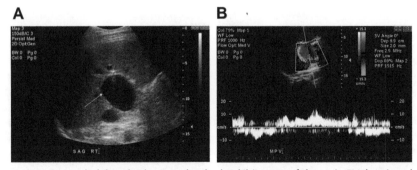

Fig. 15. PV aneurysm. Grayscale (*A*) and color Doppler duplex (*B*) images of the main PV showing abnormal aneurysmal dilatation of the PV at the hilum (*arrow* in *A*) with internal to-and-fro flow (yin-yang appearance) and disorganized flow on color Doppler duplex, which emphasizes the importance of evaluating all cystic-appearing lesions with Doppler in the posttransplant ultrasound examination. ([A] *Modified from* Friedewald SM, Molmenti EP, DeJong MB, et al. Vascular and nonvascular complications of liver transplants: sonographic evaluation and correlation with other imaging modalities and findings at surgery and pathology. Ultrasound Quarterly 2003;19:83; with permission.)

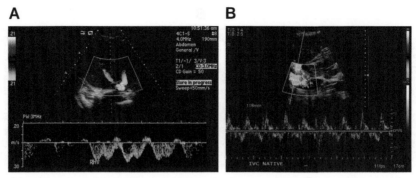

Fig. 16. Normal hepatic vein and IVC. Color Doppler duplex images of the right hepatic vein (*A*) and the IVC (*B*) showing normal venous flow with triphasic waveforms, reflecting variations in the cardiac cycle. The phasicity is often more pronounced in the IVC because of the closer proximity to the heart (*B*).

IVC and Hepatic Vein Complications

IVC and hepatic vein complications occur in approximately 1% to 2.4% of cadaveric whole-liver transplantations and include stenosis and thrombosis.[54,65,66] However, hepatic vein complications are more common with LDLT as a result

of hepatic vein anastomoses and venous reconstructions.[67]

IVC stenosis most often occurs at the anastomotic sites.[54,68] Causes in the early postoperative period may relate to size discrepancy of the donor and recipient vena cava, supracaval kinking from

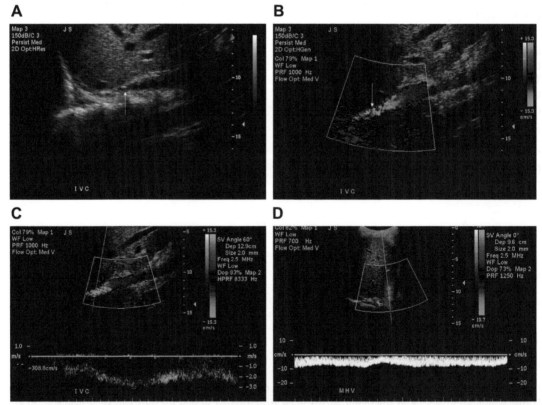

Fig. 17. IVC stenosis. (*A*) Grayscale image of the IVC showing focal area of narrowing of the IVC (*arrow*). (*B*) Color Doppler image at the same level showing associated aliasing at the site of narrowing (*arrow*). (*C*) Color Doppler duplex image showing markedly increased IVC velocity (309 cm/s/s) at the site of narrowing. (*D*) Color Doppler duplex image of the middle hepatic vein shows associated decreased pulsatility with a monophasic intrahepatic venous waveform.

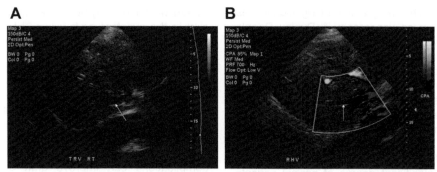

Fig. 18. HVT. (*A*) Grayscale image of the right hepatic vein shows subtle intraluminal echoes (*arrow*). (*B*) Power Doppler image of the right hepatic vein shows absence of flow, compatible with hepatic vein thrombosis (*arrow*). ([*B*] *From* Friedewald SM, Molmenti EP, DeJong MB, et al. Vascular and nonvascular complications of liver transplants: sonographic evaluation and correlation with other imaging modalities and findings at surgery and pathology. Ultrasound Quarterly 2003;19:82; with permission.)

liver rotation, or compression from adjacent hematoma or edematous liver.[66] Delayed stenosis may occur secondary to chronic thrombosis, fibrosis, or intimal hyperplasia.[10] As with other vessels, IVC stenosis can lead to thrombosis.[66]

With IVC stenosis, grayscale imaging may reveal vessel narrowing with or without associated thrombus (**Fig. 17**A).[69] Occasionally, size discrepancy may cause apparent focal narrowing on grayscale images without associated functional

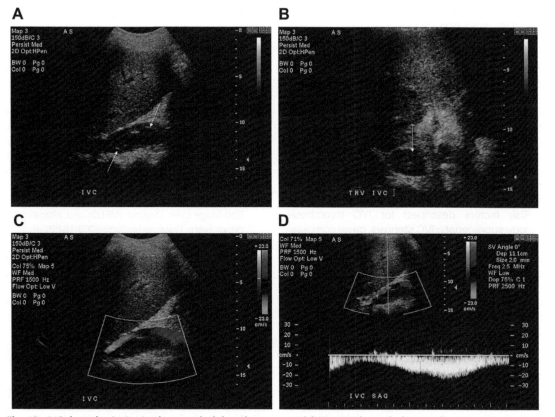

Fig. 19. IVC thrombosis. Sagittal grayscale (*A*) and transverse (*B*) images through the IVC showing echogenic intraluminal thrombus (*arrows*). Color Doppler (*C*) and color Doppler duplex (*D*) images showing flow around the thrombus, indicating that the thrombus is nonocclusive.

stenosis, as shown by a lack of significant pressure gradient on venography.[69] Duplex Doppler may show a threefold or fourfold increase in velocity measurements across the stenotic IVC segment (see **Fig. 17**B, C).[10]

Qualitative changes in hepatic vein and IVC waveforms have been reported with IVC and hepatic vein stenoses, with decreased phasicity and monophasic waveforms reported (see **Fig. 17**D).[67,69] Although sensitive, this finding is not specific, with monophasic waveforms also seen in a significant degree of normal patients, particularly in the early postoperative setting.[67]

Chong and colleagues[51] use the venous pulsatility index, a quantitative measure of venous phasicity, as a parameter to aid in the detection of venous outflow obstruction. Venous pulsatility index is calculated from the difference between the maximum and minimum frequency shifts in the venous waveform divided by the maximum.[70] Chong and colleagues[51] report that lower mean pulsatility indices (calculated by averaging the hepatic veins and IVC) are associated with an increased risk of outflow vein stenoses, with a venous pulsatility index of less than 0.45 achieving greater than a 95% specificity for venous stenosis. Normal outflow veins were found to show a mean venous pulsatility index of 0.75.[51]

Balloon angioplasty with or without stent placement is the treatment of choice in symptomatic hepatic vein or IVC stenosis; however, surgical correction is also a treatment option.[46,67,68]

The appearance of hepatic vein or IVC thrombosis is similar to that of PVT. Grayscale images typically show intraluminal echogenic thrombus (**Fig. 18**A, **Fig. 19**A, B), but can appear near normal if the thrombus is acute and anechoic or hypoechoic. Doppler imaging shows no or decreased intraluminal flow, depending on the degree of thrombosis (see **Fig. 18**B, **Fig. 19**C, D).[10]

Risk factors described for IVC thrombosis include suprahepatic IVC stenosis, caval compression by the liver, and hypercoagulable states.[66,68] Hepatic vein thromboses can also be seen in the setting of IVC stenosis, IVC thrombosis, or hypercoagulable states.[59] As mentioned previously, LDLT is a risk factor for hepatic vein thrombosis because of the hepatic venous anastomoses and venous reconstructions.[67] Presentation of IVC occlusion may include abdominal pain, ascites, lower extremity edema, liver dysfunction, and/or renal dysfunction.[54,68]

Treatment of IVC thrombosis depends on the location, with suprahepatic IVC thrombosis usually treated with thrombectomy via a right atrial approach and infrahepatic thrombosis usually treated with thrombectomy via cavostomy.[66]

Retransplantation may be needed with IVC occlusion in the event of graft failure.[68] Hepatic vein thromboses can be treated with local thrombolytic therapy.[71]

SUMMARY

Duplex Doppler ultrasound is an important diagnostic tool in the postoperative liver transplant for the diagnosis of vascular complications, suspected or unsuspected. Early diagnosis of vascular complications can improve graft and patient survival by allowing earlier treatment. Because of the range of normal appearances in the immediate postoperative liver transplant duplex Doppler ultrasound, the ability to distinguish normal postoperative findings from true complications is critical for interpretation. Duplex Doppler ultrasound can triage patients in whom further diagnostic studies are clinically indicated, emergent surgical intervention is required, or in which serial duplex ultrasound examinations should be performed.

ACKNOWLEDGMENTS

The authors thank Geri Mancini for the diagrams in **Figs. 1** and **2** and Ms Sharon Ritter for assistance with manuscript preparation.

REFERENCES

1. Starzl TE, Groth CG, Brettschneider L, et al. Orthotopic homotransplantations of the human liver. Ann Surg 1968;168:392–414.
2. O'Leary JG, Lepe R, Davis GL. Indications for liver transplantation. Gastroenterology 2008;134:1764–76.
3. Malinchoc M, Kamath PS, Gordon FD, et al. A model to predict poor survival in patients undergoing transjugular intrahepatic portosystemic shunts. Hepatology 2000;31:864–71.
4. Wiesner R, Edwards E, Freeman R, et al. Model for End-Stage Liver Disease (MELD) and allocation of donor livers. Gastroenterology 2003;124:91–6.
5. Mazzaferro V, Regalia E, Doci R, et al. Liver transplantation for the treatment of small hepatocellular carcinomas in patients with cirrhosis. N Engl J Med 1996;334:693–9.
6. Renz JF, Yersiz H, Farmer DG, et al. Changing faces of liver transplantation: partial-liver grafts for adults. J Hepatobiliary Pancreat Surg 2003;10:31–44.
7. Middleton PF, Duffield M, Lynch SV, et al. Living donor liver transplantation-adult donor outcomes: a systematic review. Liver Transpl 2006;12:24–30.
8. Lee SG. Living-donor liver transplantation in adults. Br Med Bull 2010;94:33–48.
9. Mehrabi A, Fonouni H, Muller SA, et al. Current concepts in transplant surgery: liver transplantation today. Langenbecks Arch Surg 2008;393:245–60.

10. Crossin JD, Muradali D, Wilson SR. US of liver trans-plants: normal and abnormal. Radiographics 2003; 23:1093–114.

11. Starzl ET, Marchioro TL, Von Kaulla KN, et al. Homo-transplantation of the liver in humans. Surg Gynecol Obstet 1963;117:659–76.

12. Tzakis A, Todo S, Starzl TE. Orthotopic liver trans-plantation with preservation of the inferior vena cava. Ann Surg 1989;210(5):649–52.

13. Belghiti J, Panis Y, Sauvanet A, et al. A new tech-nique of side to side caval anastomosis during or-thotopic hepatic transplantation without inferior vena caval occlusion. Surg Gynecol Obstet 1992; 175:270–2.

14. Burdick JF, Pitt HA, Colombani PM, et al. Superior mesenteric vein inflow for liver transplantation when the portal vein is occluded. Surgery 1990; 107:342–5.

15. Merion RM, Burtch GD, Ham JM, et al. The hepatic artery in liver transplantation. Transplantation 1989; 48:438–43.

16. Melada E, Maggi U, Rossi G, et al. Back-table arte-rial reconstructions in liver transplantation: single-center experience. Transplant Proc 2005;37(6): 2587–8.

17. Shaw BW, Iwatsuki S, Starzl TE. Alternative methods of arterialization of the hepatic graft. Surg Gynecol Obstet 1984;159:490–3.

18. Bismuth H. Surgical anatomy and anatomical surgery of the liver. World J Surg 1982;6:3–9.

19. Nagasue N, Yukaya H, Ogawa Y, et al. Human liver regeneration after major hepatic resection. A study of normal liver and livers with chronic hepatitis and cirrhosis. Ann Surg 1987;206:30–9.

20. Broelsch CE, Emond JC, Thistlethwaite JR, et al. Liver transplantation with reduced-size donor organs. Transplantation 1988;45:519–23.

21. Pichlmayr R, Ring B, Gubervatis G, et al. [Transplanta-tion of a donor liver to 2 recipients (splitting transplan-tation) - a new method in the further development of segmental liver transplantation]. Langenbecks Archiv fur Chirurgie 1988;373:127–30 [in German].

22. Busuttil RW, Goss JA. Split liver transplantation. Ann Surg 1999;229:313–21.

23. Strong RW, Lynch SV, Ong TH, et al. Successful liver transplantation from a living donor to her son. N Engl J Med 1990;21:1505–7.

24. Hashikura Y, Makuuchi M, Kawasaki S, et al. Successful living-related partial liver transplantation to an adult patient. Lancet 1994;343:1233–4.

25. Kiuchi T, Kasahar M, Uryuhara K, et al. Impact of graft size mismatching on graft prognosis in liver transplantation from living donors. Transplantation 1999;67:321–7.

26. Lo CM, Fan ST, Liu CL, et al. Adult-to-adult living donor transplantation using extended right lobe grafts. Ann Surg 1997;226:261–9.

27. Fan ST, Lo CM, Liu CL, et al. Safety of donors in liver donor liver transplantation using right lobe grafts. Arch Surg 2000;135:336–40.

28. Hwang S, Lee SG, Sung KB, et al. Long-term inci-dence, risk factors, and management of biliary complications after adult living donor liver transplan-tation. Liver Transpl 2006;12:831–8.

29. Lee S-G. Techniques of reconstruction of hepatic veins in living-donor liver transplantation, especially for right hepatic vein and major short hepatic veins of right-lobe graft. J Hepatobiliary Pancreat Surg 2006;13:131–8.

30. Langnas AN, Marujo W, Stratta RJ, et al. Vascular complications after orthotopic liver transplantation. Am J Surg 1991;161:76–82.

31. Garcia-Criado A, Gilabert R, Berzigotti A, et al. Doppler ultrasound findings in the hepatic artery shortly after liver transplantation. AJR Am J Roent-genol 2009;193:128–35.

32. Brody MB, Rodgers SK, Horrow MM. Spectrum of normal or near-normal sonographic findings after or-thotopic liver transplantation. Ultrasound Q 2008;24: 257–65.

33. Garcia-Criado A, Gilabert R, Salmeron JM, et al. Significance of and contributing factors for a high resistive index on Doppler sonography of the hepatic artery immediately after surgery: prognostic implications for liver transplant recipients. AJR Am J Roentgenol 2003;181:831–8.

34. Strange BJ, Glanemann M, Nuessler NC, et al. Hepatic artery thrombosis after adult liver transplan-tation. Liver Transpl 2003;9:612–20.

35. Wozney P, Zajko AB, Bron KM, et al. Vascular compli-cations after liver transplantation: a 5-year experi-ence. AJR Am J Roentgenol 1986;147:657–63.

36. Duffy JP, Hong JC, Famer DG, et al. Vascular complications of orthotopic liver transplantation: experience in more than 4,200 patients. J Am Coll Surg 2009;208:896–905.

37. Silva MA, Jambulingam PS, Gunson BK, et al. Hepatic artery thrombosis following orthotopic liver transplan-tation: a 10-year experience from a single centre in the United Kingdom. Liver Transpl 2006;12:146–51.

38. Bhattacharjya S, Gunson BK, Mirza DF, et al. De-layed hepatic artery thrombosis in adult orthotopic liver transplantation-a 12-year experience. Trans-plantation 2001;71(11):1592–6.

39. Bekker J, Ploem S, de Jong KP. Early hepatic artery thrombosis after liver transplantation: a systemic review of the incidence, outcomes and risk factors. Am J Transplant 2009;9:746–57.

40. Tzakis AG, Gordon RD, Shaw BW, et al. Clinical presentation of hepatic artery thrombosis after liver transplantation in the cyclosporine era. Transplanta-tion 1985;40(6):667–71.

41. Dodd GD III, Memel DS, Zajko AB, et al. Hepa-tic artery stenosis and thrombosis in transplant

recipients: Doppler diagnosis with resistive index and systolic acceleration time. Radiology 1994;192: 657–61.

42. Nolten A, Sproat IA. Hepatic artery thrombosis after liver transplantation: temporal accuracy of diagnosis with duplex US and the syndrome of impending thrombosis. Radiology 1996;198:53–559.

43. Singhal A, Stokes K, Sebastian A, et al. Endovascular treatment of hepatic artery thrombosis following liver transplantation. Transpl Int 2010;23: 245–56.

44. Abbasoglu O, Levy MF, Vodapally MS, et al. Hepatic artery stenosis after liver transplantation-incidence, presentation, treatment, and long term outcome. Transplantation 1997;63:250–5.

45. Dravid VS, Shapiro MJ, Needleman L, et al. Arterial abnormalities following orthotopic liver transplantation: arteriographic findings and correlation with Doppler sonographic findings. AJR Am J Roentgenol 1994;163:585–98.

46. Raby N, Karani J, Thomas S, et al. Stenoses of vascular anastomoses after hepatic transplantation: treatment with balloon angioplasty. AJR Am J Roentgenol 1991;157:167–71.

47. Marshall MM, Muiesan P, Srinivasan P, et al. Hepatic artery pseudoaneurysms following liver transplantation: incidence, presenting features and management. Clin Radiol 2001;56:579–87.

48. Strange B, Settmacher U, Glanemann M, et al. Aneurysms of the hepatic artery after liver transplantation. Transplant Proc 2000;32:533–4.

49. Zajko AB, Tobben PJ, Eszuivel CO, et al. Pseudoaneurysms following orthotopic liver transplantation: clinical and radiologic manifestations. Transplant Proc 1989;21:2457–9.

50. Rosenthal SJ, Harrison LA, Baxter KG, et al. Doppler US of helical flow in the portal vein. Radiographics 1995;15:1103–11.

51. Chong WK, Beland JC, Weeks SM. Sonographic evaluation of venous obstruction in liver transplants. AJR Am J Roentgenol 2007;188:W515–21.

52. Friedewald SM, Molmeni EP, DeJong R, et al. Vascular and nonvascular complications of liver transplants: sonographic evaluation and correlation with other imaging modalities and findings at surgery and pathology. Ultrasound Q 2003;19:71–85.

53. Stell D, Downey D, Marotta P, et al. Prospective evaluation of the role of quantitative Doppler ultrasound surveillance in liver transplantation. Liver Transpl 2004;10:1183–8.

54. Settmacher U, Nussler NC, Glanemann M, et al. Venous complications after orthotopic liver transplantation. Clin Transplant 2000;14:235–41.

55. Lee J, Ben-Ami T, Yousefzadeh D, et al. Extrahepatic portal vein stenosis in recipients of living-donor allografts: Doppler sonography. AJR Am J Roentgenol 1996;167:85–90.

56. Kyoden Y, Tamura S, Sugawara Y, et al. Portal vein complications after adult-to-adult living donor liver transplantation. Transpl Int 2008;21:1136–44.

57. Huang TL, Cheng YF, Chen TY, et al. Doppler ultrasound evaluation of postoperative portal vein stenosis in adult living donor liver transplantation. Transplant Proc 2010;42:879–81.

58. Mullan CP, Siewert B, Kane RA, et al. Can Doppler sonography discern between hemodynamically significant and insignificant portal vein stenosis after adult liver transplantation? AJR 2010;195:1438–43.

59. Glockner JF, Forauer AR. Vascular or ischemic complications after liver transplantation. AJR 1999; 173:1055–9.

60. Scantlebury VP, Zajko AB, Esquivel CO, et al. Successful reconstruction of late portal vein stenosis after hepatic transplantation. Arch Surg 1989;124:503–5.

61. di Francesco F, Gruttadauria S, Caruso S, et al. Huge extrahepatic portal vein aneurysm as a late complication of liver transplantation. World J Hepatol 2010;2:201–2.

62. Ferraz-Neto BH, Sakabe D, Buttros DA, et al. Portal vein aneurysm as late complication of liver transplantation: a case report. Transplant Proc 2004;36:970–1.

63. Koc Z, Oguzkurt L, Ulusan S. Portal venous system aneurysms: imaging, clinical findings, and a possible new etiologic factor. AJR Am J Roentgenol 2007; 189:1023–30.

64. Jequier S, Jequler JC, Hanqulnet S, et al. Orthotopic liver transplants in children: change in hepatic venous Doppler wave pattern as an indicator of acute rejection. Radiology 2003;227:105–12.

65. Lerut J, Tzakis AG, Bron K, et al. Complications of venous reconstruction in human orthotopic liver transplantation. Ann Surg 1987;205:404–14.

66. Brouwers MA, De Jong KP, Peeters PM, et al. Inferior vena caval obstruction after orthotopic liver transplantation. Clin Transplant 2004;8:9–22.

67. Ko EY, Kim TK, Kim PN, et al. Hepatic vein stenosis after living donor liver transplantation: evaluation with Doppler US. Radiology 2003;229:806–10.

68. Pfammatter T, Williams DM, Lane KL, et al. Suprahepatic caval anastomotic stenosis complicating orthotopic liver transplantation: treatment with percutaneous transluminal angioplasty, wallstent placement, or both. AJR Am J Roentgenol 1997;168:477–80.

69. Rossi AR, Pozniak MA, Zarvan NP. Upper inferior vena caval anastomotic stenosis in liver transplant recipients: Doppler us diagnosis. Radiology 1993; 187:387–9.

70. Coulden RA, Lomas DJ, Farman P, et al. Doppler ultrasound of the hepatic veins: normal appearances. Clin Radiol 1992;25:223–7.

71. Lopez-Benitez R, Barragan-Campos HM, Richter GM, et al. Interventional radiologic procedures in the treatment of complications after liver transplantation. Clin Transplant 2009;23:92–101.

A Pot Pourri of Abdominal Doppler Cases

Gaurav Vij, MD[a],*, Ulrike M. Hamper, MD, MBA[b],
M. Robert De Jong, RDMS, RVT[b], Leslie M. Scoutt, MD[a]

KEYWORDS

• Abdomen • Doppler • Artery • Vein

CASE 1: MEDIAN ARCUATE LIGAMENT SYNDROME

The median arcuate ligament is a fibrous band that passes over the abdominal aorta above the level of the celiac axis in most individuals and connects the right and left diaphragmatic crura on either side of the aortic hiatus. However, in approximately 10% to 24% of people, the ligament inserts more inferiorly and crosses over the proximal portion of the celiac axis causing compression of the proximal celiac axis, which is more pronounced in expiration.[1] Although this congenital variant seems to be an incidental finding in many patients, between 87% and 50% of patients with visible compression of the proximal celiac axis present with pain, nausea, vomiting, and/or weight loss,[2,3] a constellation of findings described first in 1963 by Harjola.[4] Clinically significant compression of the celiac axis is termed median arcuate ligament syndrome (MALS), although this is a controversial clinical entity. Most cases have been described in thin women between the ages of 20 and 40 years. Pain may or may not be associated with eating. On physical examination a midepigastric bruit that varies with respiration may be heard.[1]

The pathophysiology of MALS is not yet fully established. Some investigators think that compression of the celiac axis results in distal ischemia causing abdominal pain despite the well-known fact that narrowing of 2 of the 3 mesenteric vessels is required to induce mesenteric ischemia. Others suggest that steal from collaterals from the superior mesenteric artery causes the abdominal pain. Compression or ischemia of the celiac ganglion has also been postulated as the cause of abdominal pain in patients with MALS.[5,6]

The diagnosis of MALS is most often made with conventional angiography or with three-dimensional computed tomographic angiography (CTA) by the demonstration of focal narrowing of the proximal celiac axis, typically 5 mm from the origin, which becomes more pronounced on expiration. In addition, a characteristic fishhook appearance of the proximal celiac axis on expiration is observed.[1] The presence of poststenotic dilatation and/or collaterals to the distal celiac bed from the superior mesenteric artery increases the specificity of the angiographic or CTA findings, which can help distinguish this condition from other causes of celiac artery narrowing, such as atherosclerosis.[1] Duplex Doppler ultrasound (US) can be used as a less expensive alternative screening test. The following US criteria have been used to diagnose MALS on US: (1) variation of peak systolic velocity (PSV) in the celiac axis during respiration with an increase in PSV during expiration to greater than 200 cm/s; (2) a greater than 3:1 ratio of PSV in the celiac artery in expiration compared with the PSV in the abdominal aorta immediately below the diaphragm; and (3) a fishhook appearance of the configuration of the celiac axis on color Doppler

[a] Department of Diagnostic Radiology, Yale University School of Medicine, 333 Cedar Street, PO Box 208042, New Haven, CT 06520-8042, USA
[b] Ultrasound Section, Russell H. Morgan Department of Radiology and Radiological Science, The Johns Hopkins University, School of Medicine, 600 North Wolfe Street, Room B-106, Baltimore, MD 21287, USA
* Corresponding author.
E-mail address: gaurav.vij@yale.edu

Ultrasound Clin 6 (2011) 531–550
doi:10.1016/j.cult.2011.07.005
1556-858X/11/$ – see front matter © 2011 Elsevier Inc. All rights reserved.

Case 1. This 34-year-old woman presented with abdominal pain and weight loss. Color Doppler images of the celiac axis in inspiration (*A*) and expiration (*B*) show a change in appearance of the celiac axis. During expiration, the celiac axis becomes more acutely curved toward the head, developing a fishhook configuration. Note that the peak systolic velocity (PSV) also increases from 118 cm/s in inspiration (*C*) to 232 cm/s in expiration (*D*). This patient had median arcuate ligament syndrome that was surgically treated with relief of symptoms. (*Reprinted from* Scoutt LM. Ultrasound: Vascular. In Approach to Diagnosis: a Case-Based Imaging Review. In: Baumgarten DA, Bhalla S, Salkowski LR, et al, editors. Reston (VA): ARRS; 2010. p. 11–28; with permission.)

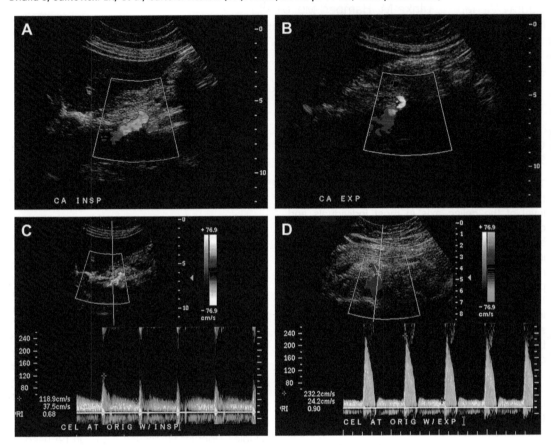

or grayscale imaging during expiration.[7,8] Some investigators have suggested that the specificity of these findings is increased when the US examination is performed in the erect position.[8] However, the specificity of these US findings in the celiac axis is controversial because such findings can be seen in asymptomatic patients or in patients with celiac stenosis caused by atherosclerosis.

Laparoscopic surgery with division or resection of the median arcuate ligament to relieve the compression of the proximal duodenum is considered by most to be the treatment of choice for patients with MALS.[6] In some patients, the ligamentous constriction of the celiac axis causes vascular damage, which may require vascular reconstruction.[6] In others, decompression, division, resection, or neurolysis of the fibrotic celiac ganglion has proven to be of benefit.[6] However, because the CTA and US findings are nonspecific, surgical decompression may not always result in a durable relief of symptoms.[1,5,6] Reilly and colleagues[9] reported that patients between the ages of 40 and 60 years who present with postprandial pain and a greater than 9-kg weight loss with poststenotic dilatation and collateral vessels on angiography or CTA respond best to surgery.

CASE 2: OVARIAN TORSION

Case 2. A 24-year-old woman presents to the emergency room with intermittent left pelvic pain. Grayscale images (*A, B*) show that the left ovary is enlarged with heterogeneous central stroma and peripheral displacement of small follicles. Note small amount of adjacent free fluid (*asterisk* in *B*). Color Doppler image (*C*) shows color flow in the ovarian parenchyma with arterial flow confirmed on a spectral Doppler tracing (*D*). Torsion of the left ovary was found at laparoscopy.

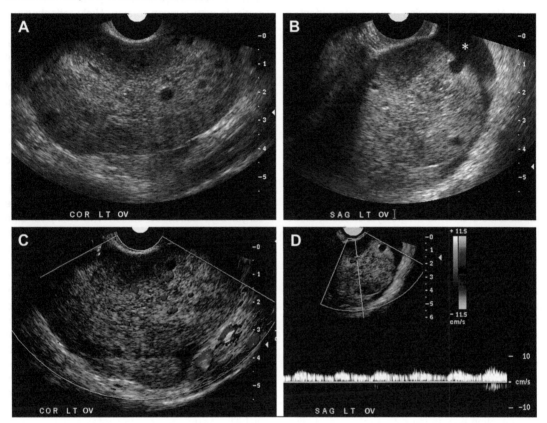

Ovarian torsion accounts for approximately 2.7% of all gynecologic operative emergencies.[10] Ovarian torsion occurs most commonly on the right, likely because there is less space in the left adnexa for the ovary to twist because of the presence of the sigmoid colon. Classically, patients with ovarian torsion present with sudden onset of severe pelvic pain often accompanied by rebound tenderness. However, in as many as 50% of all cases, adnexal torsion may be partial or intermittent, presenting with mild or intermittent symptoms that may mimic other pelvic disorders.[11]

Adnexal torsion is most common in women of reproductive age, but has been reported in all age groups. An underlying ovarian mass is found in 50% to 80% of cases.[10,12] These masses are most commonly benign and it is thought that inflammation, adhesions, or local invasion by malignant lesions prevents twisting of the ovarian pedicle.[10,12] Up to

20% of cases are associated with pregnancy, most commonly occurring in the first trimester or post partum.[13] Patients undergoing ovulation induction are also at increased risk of developing ovarian torsion.[14] Prior pelvic surgery, especially tubal ligation, is also a risk factor for ovarian torsion.[15] In children with ovarian torsion, the underlying ovary is more often normal and laxity of the ovarian ligaments and sudden change in intra-abdominal pressure have been postulated as mechanisms for ovarian torsion in the pediatric patient population.[16,17]

Adnexal torsion may involve the ovary, fallopian tube, or both. As the adnexal pedicle twists, lymphatic obstruction occurs, resulting in the development of ovarian edema and enlargement. Further twisting of the ovarian pedicle leads to venous and arterial obstruction. Once arterial obstruction occurs, ovarian necrosis results quickly unless surgical decompression is performed. Early intervention has been shown to decrease the rate of complications such as peritonitis and pulmonary embolus, and increase the rate of ovarian salvage.[18,19] However, it should be remembered that, because the ovary has a dual blood supply, torsion of one arterial system may be masked or compensated for by increased flow in the other artery. Also, ovarian torsion may be intermittent or partial in many cases, preserving blood flow at least intermittently. Furthermore, both venous and arterial collateral flow may develop in cases of chronic adnexal torsion.[18]

In a patient suspected of having ovarian torsion, ultrasound is considered the imaging modality of choice. An enlarged ovary with an ill-defined and heterogeneous central ovarian stroma and peripheral displacement of the small ovarian follicles (Fig. 2) is the most characteristic grayscale US appearance, but is not always present.[18–21] Once necrosis has occurred, the grayscale US appearance is highly variable and sometimes mimics the appearance of a hemorrhagic cyst or sac of blood if the parenchyma has completely liquefied. An underlying ovarian mass is commonly observed and may obscure visualization of the ovarian parenchyma. A small amount of adjacent free pelvic fluid is often present. The enlarged ovary is often tender on examination and found in an atypical, midline position. Careful search between the ovary and the uterus may reveal an enlarged, edematous fallopian tube that, on cross section, may have a targetlike appearance of alternating hypoechoic and echogenic rings with the hypoechoic rings representing twisted or swirling vessels within the swollen pedicle.[22] In addition, grayscale US evaluation has an important role in excluding other causes of abdominal and pelvic pain such as a ruptured or hemorrhagic cyst, tubo-ovarian abscess, appendicitis, and ureteral calculi.

Although it was initially postulated that absence of flow on Doppler interrogation would be a sensitive and specific finding of ovarian torsion, color and spectral Doppler findings are variable in patients with ovarian torsion, likely reflecting the degree of torquing and tension on the twisted ovarian pedicle, chronicity or intermittent nature, and the presence of a dual blood supply to the ovary. Lack of venous and arterial flow in an adnexal mass is consistent with the diagnosis of ovarian torsion.[23] However, if the ovary is deep to the US beam, Doppler flow may not be demonstrable in a normal ovary, leading to false-positive diagnoses based on Doppler findings alone. On color Doppler interrogation the vessels in the twisted ovarian pedicle will light up with color (unless thrombosed) creating the so-called "whirlpool sign", ie the color Doppler equivalent of the target sign described earlier. The whirlpool sign has also been reported as a specific finding of ovarian torsion.[22,24] However, arterial and venous ovarian flow have been documented on Doppler US interrogation in many cases of surgically proved ovarian torsion (see Fig. 2).[18,21] In cases of intermittent torsion or torsion/detorsion, blood flow may be transiently increased. Hence, in a patient with grayscale features suggestive of ovarian torsion or strong clinical concern, the presence of blood flow to the ovary on Doppler interrogation should not prevent the diagnosis of ovarian torsion. Whether the presence of both arterial and venous intra-ovarian flow is predictive of ovarian viability at surgery remains controversial.[18,23–25]

CASE 3: ARTERIOVENOUS FISTULA AND PSEUDOANEURYSM IN A RENAL TRANSPLANT

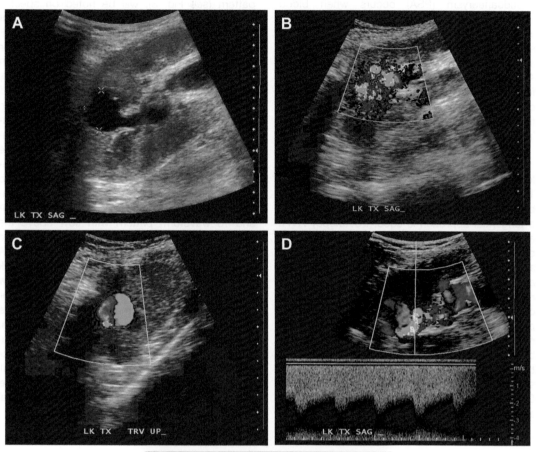

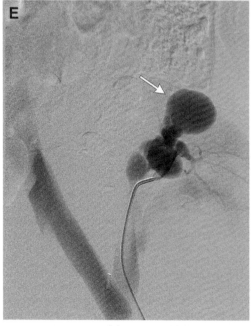

An arteriovenous fistula (AVF) is an abnormal direct communication between an artery and a vein. A pseudoaneurysm (PSA) occurs when blood extravasates through a tear in an arterial wall and is contained by a pseudocapsule of compressed surrounding soft tissues. Both AVFs and PSAs are known complications of renal biopsy. Although AVFs and PSAs are both common complications following percutaneous biopsy, they are usually diagnosed independently and it is uncommon to find an AVF and PSA adjacent to each other as in this patient.

The reported incidence of AVFs following renal biopsy is estimated at 0.3% to 19% in the native kidney and 6% to 8% in renal transplants.[26–30] The incidence of clinically significant AVFs after biopsy is significantly lower if US guidance with a tangential approach is used. Postbiopsy AVFs are most commonly asymptomatic and are incidental findings. However, large AVFs may occasionally cause flank pain, gross hematuria, hypertension, arterial bruits, congestive heart failure, and, rarely, renal insufficiency.[26–37] Although symptoms most commonly occur in the immediate postbiopsy period, delayed presentation has also been reported.[33–35] Most clinically significant AVFs can be diagnosed on Doppler US. Increased flow through the AVF results in vibration of the surrounding soft tissues that will appear on color Doppler US as a focal color mosaic overlying the adjacent soft tissues, called a soft tissue bruit

(Fig. 3). Increased peak systolic and end diastolic velocities, a so-called low-resistance waveform pattern (see Fig. 3), will be noted on spectral Doppler tracings of the feeding artery and the draining vein will show increased velocity of flow with a pulsatile waveform.[26,29] Small AVFs may resolve spontaneously. However, AVFs that are symptomatic, extremely large, or extrarenal are usually treated with percutaneous embolization.[32–34,37]

On grayscale imaging, a PSA appears as an anechoic round or saccular cystic structure adjacent to an artery that fills in with color in a yin-yang pattern on color Doppler interrogation (see Fig. 3). Thrombus within the PSA appears hypoechoic on grayscale imaging and as a color void on color flow imaging. Spectral Doppler interrogation of the neck of a PSA classically reveals a to-and-fro waveform pattern with flow above the baseline heading toward the PSA in systole and below the baseline heading away from the PSA during diastole, if the neck is narrow. If the neck is wide, a more irregular disorganized blood flow pattern is observed.[26,29] Most PSAs are asymptomatic. A small PSA may be watched to see whether it undergoes spontaneous thrombosis. However, because of the risk of rupture, PSAs greater than 2 cm in diameter and enlarging or extrarenal PSAs are typically treated with percutaneous embolization. Stent placement may be a preferred method of treatment of extrarenal PSAs.

Case 3. This 73-year-old male status post renal transplant presented with hematuria following percutaneous renal biopsy for increasing creatinine level. (A) Grayscale image of the transplanted kidney shows an anechoic round structure (calipers) in the renal cortex at the upper pole. In a patient status post renal biopsy, this most likely represents either a pseudoaneurysm (PSA) or a focally distended draining vein from an arteriovenous fistula (AVF). Note tubular anechoic structure leading to this area from the echogenic renal sinus, likely representing either a distended feeding artery or draining vein. (B) Color Doppler image shows focal color aliasing indicating high-velocity flow at this site as well as surrounding red and blue speckles that indicate a soft tissue bruit caused by tissue vibration. The red and blue color coding indicates lower-velocity flow, typical of a soft tissue bruit. This constellation of findings could be seen with either an AVF or PSA. (C) Color Doppler image after increasing the color scale and wall filter. The soft tissue bruit is no longer present and alternating red and blue flow, the so-called yin-yang color flow pattern typical of a PSA, is observed. (D) Spectral Doppler tracing does not reveal the high-velocity to-and-fro waveform pattern classically found in the neck of a PSA but rather a low-resistance waveform pattern with increased systolic and diastolic flow, which is diagnostic of an AVF. (E) Angiogram shows both the outpouching of a PSA (arrow) as well as a tangle of vessels inferiorly with early venous drainage diagnostic of an AVF. (Reprinted from Piyasena RV, Hamper UM. Doppler ultrasound evaluation of renal transplants. Appl Radiol 2010;39:31; with permission.)

CASE 4: AIR IN THE PORTAL VEIN

Case 4. A 54-year-old patient status post renal transplantation presented with abdominal pain. (*A*) Grayscale image of the main portal vein shows punctuate echogenic foci within the vessel lumen. Although these could be artifactual in nature, on real-time imaging they could be seen to move peripherally. (*B*) Grayscale image of the liver shows echogenic foci in the liver parenchyma extending to the liver capsule in a predominantly linear configuration. No dirty shadowing or ring-down artifact is seen. Some of the echogenic foci are in a more geographic configuration consistent with extension into the smaller, closely branching distal portal venules. (*C, D*) Spectral Doppler waveforms obtained from the main portal vein show sharp, spikelike artifacts (*arrows*) in the Doppler tracing from the air bubbles in the portal vein. The spikes are caused by the highly reflective nature of air. (*E*) CT scan confirms the presence of air in the peripheral portal veins in the liver (*arrows*). This patient was on prednisone and had a markedly distended colon caused by fecal impaction without evidence on CT scan of bowel ischemia. The patient did well following disimpaction.

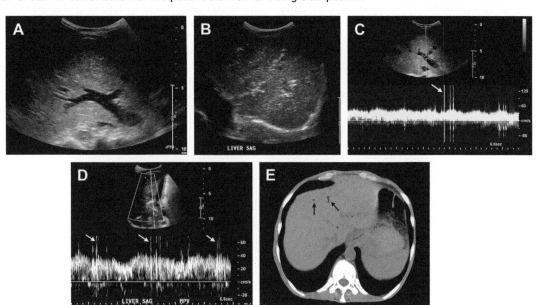

Portal venous gas is a rare, but clinically significant, radiographic finding, usually a harbinger of ischemic bowel requiring immediate surgical intervention. It was first described in 1955 by Wolfe and Evans[38] on abdominal plain radiographs in 6 neonates who died secondary to necrotic bowel. In approximately 50% of reported cases, patients with air in the portal veins also have pneumatosis intestinalis or gas within the intestinal wall.[39,40] It is generally presumed that air from the bowel wall enters the draining veins in the bowel mesentery and travels to the portal venous system[41]; thus, pneumatosis intestinalis and portal venous air likely represent progressive steps in a single process.[38] Serious, life-threatening causes include bacterial colitis/necrotizing enterocolitis, bowel ischemia/infarction (especially colon), retroperitoneal or intraperitoneal abscess, infected gallbladder, liver abscess, necrotizing pancreatitis, and bowel malignancy. The presence of air in the portal veins has also been reported in more benign processes such as bowel distention (especially stomach and colon), inflammatory bowel disease, gastric ulcer, recent interventions/surgery, and emphysema.[42] Rarely, portal or hepatic venous air may be seen on US in completely asymptomatic individuals without evidence of bowel disease, possibly because of turbulent or high-velocity blood flow.

On real-time grayscale US, highly reflective tiny foci, representing air bubbles in the portal veins, can be seen to move peripherally. Highly echogenic foci in a linear configuration with or without dirty shadowing located peripherally in the liver parenchyma can also be observed as the air in the portal venous system moves toward the liver capsule. These highly reflective foci can also be seen in scattered, less well-defined geographic areas as the air spreads into the liver parenchyma in small, branching portal venous channels.[43,44] On pulsed Doppler interrogation, spikelike signals are seen superimposed on portal venous flow pattern caused by the highly reflective nature of the portal venous air bubbles.[45,46] When air in the portal vein is diagnosed or suspected on US examination, follow-up with CT is generally recommended to evaluate for bowel disorders because this may be life threatening. However, several studies have reported that US is more sensitive than CT in detecting portal venous gas.[43,47] If portal venous air is not confirmed on follow-up CT scan, this is likely a benign or incidental finding.[48]

Air in the portal vein must be differentiated from air in the biliary tree. On grayscale images, gas within intrahepatic and extrahepatic bile ducts is seen as echogenic foci in the nondependent parts of the liver in a linear configuration within the portal triads. Posterior acoustic shadowing or ring-down artifact is often visualized, concentrated centrally near the porta hepatitis, as opposed to portal venous gas, which tends to extend to the periphery. Biliary air is often more echogenic than portal venous air, likely because it is more stationary and tends to collect rather than diffuse into the liver parenchyma. Geographic parenchymal areas of increased echogenicity are less likely to be observed in patients with air in the biliary tract. In addition, intrabiliary echogenic foci typically appear stationary, although movement can rarely be seen following change in the patient's position.

CASE 5: AORTIC DISSECTION

Case 5. This 57-year-old man presented with sudden onset of severe back pain. (*A*) Sagittal (SAG) grayscale image of the aorta (AO) shows an echogenic intraluminal flap caused by an aortic dissection. Note that the aorta is not aneurysmally dilated. (*B*) Transverse grayscale image of the aorta showing the echogenic intimal flap. Superior mesenteric artery (SMA) (*arrow*). (*C*) Transverse color Doppler image shows that both lumens are patent, although a color void caused by thrombus (*arrow*) is present in the false lumen, which is more posterior. (*D*) Spectral Doppler tracing reveals a normal high-resistance waveform pattern in the true lumen. However, note increased PSV (215 cm/s) caused by narrowing of the true lumen. (*E*) Spectral Doppler tracing of the false lumen showing an abnormal waveform pattern with decreased PSV.

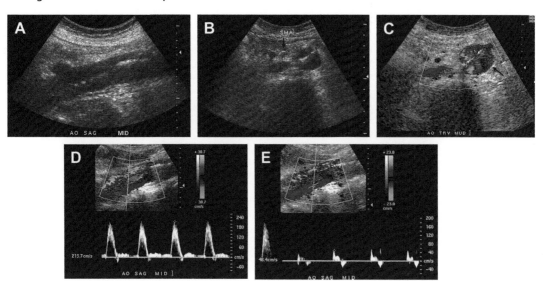

An aortic dissection begins with a tear in the intima of the aortic wall and subsequent passage of blood into the aortic media through the tear, separating the intima from the surrounding media and/or adventitia and creating a false lumen. The dissection can propagate distally and/or proximally to the initial tear, involving branch vessels and the aortic valve, which can allow blood to enter the pericardial space. This process is responsible for many of the associated clinical manifestations, including ischemia (coronary, cerebral, spinal, or visceral), aortic regurgitation, and cardiac tamponade. The false lumen may supply the branch vessels from the aorta. Thus, if the false lumen thromboses and occludes, the branch vessels may occlude also. Aortic dissections usually begin in the thoracic aorta but may extend into the abdominal aorta. Rarely, aortic dissections may be isolated to the abdominal aorta. Predisposing factors for aortic dissection include hypertension, atherosclerosis, preexisting aortic aneurysm, vasculitis, collagen vascular diseases such as Ehlers Danlos and Marfan syndromes, trauma, bicuspid aortic valves, aortic coarctation, cocaine abuse, and high-intensity weight training. Aortic dissection should be clinically suspected in a patient who has abrupt onset of thoracic or abdominal pain with a sharp, tearing, or ripping character, variation in peripheral pulses (eg, absence of a proximal extremity or carotid pulse) or difference in systolic blood pressure in the right and left arm more than 20 mm Hg, and widening of the mediastinum on chest radiograph.

In the emergency department setting, chest CT is the initial study of choice. Transesophageal echocardiography (TEE) and magnetic resonance imaging are also appropriate diagnostic imaging studies if the patient is hemodynamically stable. It is particularly important to rapidly identify acute dissections involving the ascending aorta (Stanford type A), which are considered surgical emergencies. In comparison, dissections confined to the descending aorta (Stanford type B) are more likely to be hemodynamically stable and are usually treated medically.

Although ultrasound is not the imaging modality of choice if an aortic dissection in the chest is suspected, dissections in the abdominal aorta are easily visualized on ultrasound. An echogenic intimal intraluminal flap is diagnostic of dissection on grayscale imaging. The flap may be mobile on real-time imaging. Intraluminal echoes may be present if one of the lumens is thrombosed. Color Doppler imaging is helpful to determine whether both lumens are patent. Spectral Doppler may show discrepancy in flow patterns between the true and false lumens, with decreased flow with an atypical waveform pattern in the false lumen.

In the abdomen, the origins of the celiac axis, superior mesenteric artery, and renal arteries should be carefully examined to determine whether the dissection extends into these vessels. Extension of the dissection flap into these vessels may result in stenosis or thrombosis.

CASE 6: SPLENIC ARTERY ANEURYSM

Case 6. This 40-year-old woman presented with left upper quadrant pain. (*A*) Transverse grayscale image shows an enlarged anechoic structure (*asterisk*) posterior to the pancreas and splenic vein (S). A, aorta; C, inferior vena cava. Left renal vein (*arrow*). Sagittal grayscale image (*B*) shows that this structure (*asterisk*) is continuous with the splenic artery. (*C*) Grayscale image shows that the wall of this structure (*calipers*) is echogenic, consistent with calcification. (*D*) Color Doppler flow imaging showing color fill-in of this splenic artery aneurysm (*asterisk*). (*E*) Spectral Doppler tracing showing an arterial waveform. (*F*) Contrast-enhanced CT scan showing enhancement of the splenic artery aneurysm (*asterisk*).

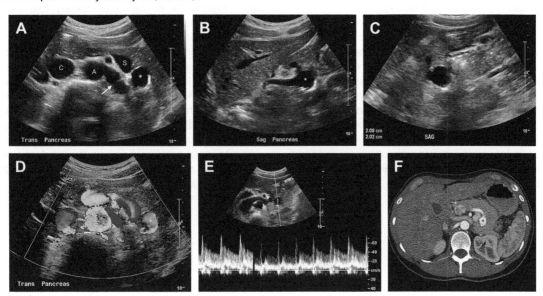

Splenic artery aneurysm (SAA) is the commonest visceral artery aneurysm. There is an association between SAAs and portal hypertension and in such patients the incidence may be as high as 7.1% compared with 1.6% in the general population. SAAs are also associated with fibromuscular dysplasia and other types of vasculitis or focal arterial inflammation, pancreatitis (often pseudoaneurysms), atherosclerosis, hypertension, autoimmune and collagen vascular disorders, intravenous drug abuse (mycotic), and trauma. SAAs are 4 times more common in women than in men and up to 95% present during pregnancy.[49] The increased incidence of symptomatic SAA in pregnancy has been postulated to be secondary to hormonal influence or shunting of blood into the splenic artery.[50] The most critical complication of SAAs is rupture, which is estimated to occur in up to 3% to 10% of cases.[50] Rupture occurring during pregnancy is associated with a disproportionately high maternal and fetal mortality. The double rupture phenomenon, first described by Brockman,[51] occurs in 20% to 25% of cases.[52,53] In this clinical scenario, patients present with sudden onset of abdominal pain, hypotension, or syncope but usually recover quickly from this initial event with

fluid resuscitation most likely secondary to the tamponade effect of the omentum or blood clot in the lesser sac surrounding the SAA. This temporary tamponade effect is believed to increase the chance of survival by providing time for diagnosis and definitive management. However, within 48 hours, this latent period is followed by free rupture into the peritoneum and abrupt onset of cardiovascular collapse. Other presenting symptoms include abdominal and back pain, the Kehr sign (pain radiating to the left shoulder caused by irritation of the diaphragm), and hemodynamic instability following rupture. Rarely, splenic infarct may occur. However, most SAAs are less than 2.5 cm in diameter and lesions of this size are usually asymptomatic and found incidentally.[53,54] Rupture is extremely rare in SAAs less than 2.5 cm.[49,53,55]

Most SAAs are solitary (71%) and saccular (80%), located in the mid or distal portion of the splenic artery (80%), frequently at the splenic hilum.[50,53,54] Surgical vascular reconstruction remains the gold standard for treatment. However, percutaneous embolization or exclusion with an intravascular stent is increasingly performed, although the durability of percutaneous therapy is not proven. Indications for treatment include symptoms/rupture, pregnancy or intent to become pregnant, increasing size, and a diameter greater than or equal to 2 cm. Asymptomatic SAAs that are less than 2 cm in diameter are either removed electively or followed closely. The risk of elective removal is extremely low and has minimal morbidity. The spleen should be preserved if possible, and splenectomy is reserved for those aneurysms found in the hilum of the spleen or during emergency situations.[50]

If an SAA is calcified, it may be seen on abdominal radiographs or CT scan. On contrast-enhanced CT, a patent SAA is visualized as an outpouching from the splenic artery. If the SAA is thrombosed and the wall is not calcified, it may be difficult to identify, mimicking lymph nodes or mesenteric veins. Although SAAs are most often diagnosed on CT scanning, US provides a noninvasive and inexpensive method of following SAAs for change in size without exposure to radiation or iodinated contrast. For these reasons, duplex Doppler US imaging is the preferred diagnostic imaging modality in pregnancy. On US, a patent SAA may be seen as an anechoic outpouching from the splenic artery on grayscale imaging that will fill in with color on color flow imaging. If calcified, the wall will be echogenic and show distal shadowing. Internal low-level echoes will be present if the SAA is thrombosed and there will be no detectable color Doppler flow. Free fluid or hemoperitoneum following rupture is also readily detected on US examination. Limitations of US examination relate to operator dependency and attenuation of sound waves secondary to obesity and/or overlying bowel gas. Hence, even in the best of hands, not all midline or central SAAs are found on US examination because of shadowing from overlying bowel gas. Heavily calcified SAA may also be difficult to detect. Although routine screening of all pregnant patients is not practical because the incidence of SAAs is low, some have suggested that screening in high-risk groups may be beneficial.[55]

CASE 7: COARCTATION OF THE AORTA PRESENTING AS RENAL ARTERY STENOSIS

Case 7. This 11-year-old boy presented with hypertension. Spectral Doppler tracings from the right (A) and left (B) main renal arteries show a dampened or tardus parvus (parvus is low velocity, tardus is delayed acceleration) waveform pattern bilaterally consistent with a proximal stenosis. The tardus parvus phenomenon is so pronounced that the waveforms almost look venous. However, note the normal left main renal vein (blue, flow heading away from the kidney) adjacent to the main renal artery (red, flow heading toward the kidney) from which the Doppler tracing was obtained (B). However, no increased velocity was noted at the origins of the renal arteries. A similar waveform is noted in the suprarenal aorta (C). Hence, the stenosis must be proximal to the abdominal aorta. The boy was subsequently found to have coarctation of the aorta. (*Reprinted from* the ARRS: Scoutt LM. Ultrasound: Vascular. In Approach to Diagnosis: a Case-Based Imaging Review. In: Baumgarten DA, Bhalla S, Salkowski LR, et al, editors. ARRS Reston (VA); 2010. p. 11–30; with permission.)

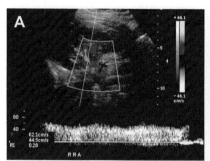

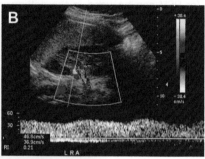

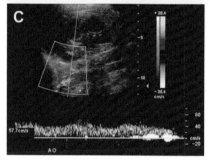

Ultrasound is frequently used in the assessment of renal artery stenosis (RAS). The kidney may be small in size and there may be an increase in echogenicity or thinning of the renal cortex, secondary to chronic ischemia.

On color Doppler interrogation, focal color aliasing in the main renal artery at the site of the stenosis is observed. Diagnostic spectral Doppler criteria for RAS (>60%) include increase of the peak systolic velocity in the main renal artery greater than or equal to 180 to 200 cm/s, ratio of the PSV in the renal artery to that in the aorta (RAR) at the level of renal arteries greater than 3.0 to 3.5, poststenotic spectral broadening,[56–58] and delayed systolic acceleration in the spectral Doppler waveforms of the segmental or interlobar arteries.[59] Delay in systolic acceleration indicates a proximal stenosis. However, it is a nonspecific finding because the precise level of the stenosis cannot be determined, just that it is more proximal

to the point of interrogation. Delay in systolic acceleration can be quantified by measuring the acceleration time (AT), which is the length of time from the onset of systole to the early systolic peak complex, or acceleration index (AI), which is the slope of the line connecting the onset of systole to the early systolic peak complex. An AT greater than 70 milliseconds and an AI less than 3 ms^2 are considered abnormal.[59] Alternatively, delay in systolic acceleration can be subjectively assessed by looking for the tardus parvus waveform, which is characterized by a slow upstroke (tardus) and low-velocity, rounded (parvus) systolic peak.[59] When renovascular hypertension is caused by atherosclerotic disease, the narrowing is found at the origin or proximal main renal artery or, more rarely, at a branch point. If the renovascular hypertension is caused by fibromuscular dysplasia, the mid to distal portion of the main renal artery is affected and a 'string-of-beads appearance may be seen.

Some investigators have suggested that, if there is diminished aortic flow (ie, depressed cardiac contractility) and PSV within the aorta is less than 40 cm/s, the RAR will be artificially increased. Conversely, in the event of substantial abdominal aortic atherosclerosis or hypertension, with PSV in the aorta greater than 100 cm/s, the RAR will be falsely depressed. In such scenarios, absolute PSV greater than 200 cm/s with poststenotic turbulence within the renal artery should be used as the primary determinant of clinically significant RAS.[60] However, whether or not the same absolute number for PSV can be used in the setting of substantially increased or decreased aortic velocity remains to be proved.

A tardus parvus waveform pattern in the intraparenchymal renal arteries is not a specific finding for stenosis of the main renal artery but may also indicate more proximal stenosis in the aorta or even at the level of the aortic valve. However, in such cases, the tardus parvus waveform is a bilateral finding in the renal arteries. Causes of narrowing of the aorta include coarctation, William syndrome, neurofibromatosis, retroperitoneal fibrosis, and some types of vasculitis. In patients with aortic coarctation, a tardus parvus waveform will be noted in the abdominal aorta as well as in the bilateral renal arteries. To diagnose coexistent stenosis of the renal artery, the PSV and RAR Doppler criteria must be used instead of relying on the intraparenchymal waveform analysis.

In conclusion, the tardus parvus waveform can be produced by a stenosis at any point proximal to the artery studied. A cause more proximal to the renal vessels in the aorta or aortic valve should be considered if bilateral tardus parvus waveforms are noted in the intraparenchymal renal arteries. Also, it is important to remember that coarctation of the aorta, neurofibromatosis, and William syndrome should be considered as possible causes of secondary hypertension, particularly in children. In adults, aortic stenosis, aortic dissections, severe atherosclerosis, and, more rarely, retroperitoneal fibrosis may cause abnormal waveforms in renal arteries.

CASE 8: ASYMMETRIC WAVEFORMS IN THE LEFT AND RIGHT HEPATIC ARTERIES

Case 8. This 54-year-old woman presented with sepsis caused by multiple liver abscesses. (*A*) Spectral Doppler tracing from the main hepatic artery (MHA) reveals a tardus parvus waveform consistent with a proximal stenosis. A similar waveform was noted in the right hepatic artery (not shown). However, a spectral tracing from the LHA (*B*) reveals a normal sharp systolic upstroke (+). Angiography showed a long segment stenosis of the common hepatic artery with a replaced left hepatic artery from the left gastric artery.

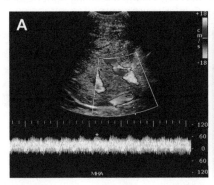 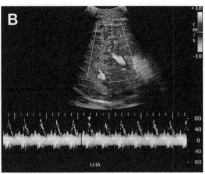

Variant hepatic artery anatomy is common, with a reported incidence of 23% to 45%.[61] In a series of 180 patients, Jones and Hardy[61] showed that the left hepatic artery had its origin from the common hepatic artery trunk in 80%, from the left gastric artery in 15%, the splenic artery in 2%, the gastroduodenal artery in 1%, and even less commonly from the aorta, celiac axis, and superior mesenteric artery (SMA). The right hepatic artery (RHA) originated from the main trunk of the common hepatic artery in 75%, the SMA in 18%, the gastroduodenal artery in 6%, and the right gastric artery or aorta in 1.6%.[61] Others have estimated the frequency of occurrence of a replaced left hepatic artery (LHA) from the left gastric artery to be 10% and that of a replaced RHA from the SMA to be 11% (Michel type II and III hepatic arterial anatomy, respectively).[62,63] These variations in anatomy can have serious implications during surgery and hence it is important for the radiologist to be aware of them.[64] Although it may be difficult to directly visualize congenital variations of the origins of the hepatic arteries, asymmetry of the intrahepatic waveforms may be a clue to their presence.

CASE 9: HEPATIC ARTERIOVENOUS MALFORMATION

Case 9. This 48-year-old woman has a history of hereditary hemorrhagic telangiectasia (HHT) and presents with right upper quadrant pain. (*A*) Color Doppler image of the right lobe of the liver shows a tangle of enlarged vessels consistent with an arteriovenous malformation. COR, coronal; RK, right kidney. More central grayscale image (*B*) shows an enlarged feeding vessel (*arrow*). Grayscale image of the porta hepatis (*C*) shows an enlarged, tortuous hepatic artery (*arrows*). G, gallbladder. (*D*) Note massively enlarged draining right hepatic vein (*arrow*) compared with the normal middle and left hepatic veins. C, inferior vena cava.

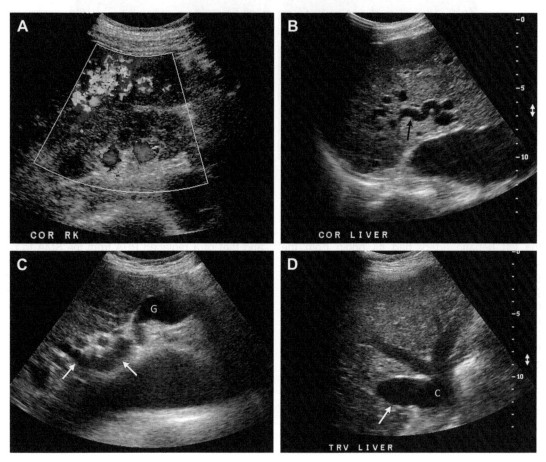

Diffuse hepatic arteriovenous malformations (AVMs) may be seen in the setting of hereditary hemorrhagic telangiectasia (HHT) or Osler-Weber-Rendu disease. The frequency of hepatic AVMs in patients with HHT has been reported to be between 8% and 31%.[65] Although often asymptomatic, liver involvement can result in high-output congestive heart failure.[66–68] Shunting of blood can rarely lead to biliary necrosis, liver abscess, and even portal hypertension.[68] Other causes of AVFs or AVMs in the liver include trauma, congenital anomaly, cirrhosis, Budd-Chiari syndrome, and neoplasms.[69–72]

The sonographic manifestations of patients with HHT and hepatic AVMs include large feeding arteries, pulsatile venous flow pattern, presence of multiple dilated tortuous tubular structures in the liver parenchyma, and large draining veins.[73–75] The dilated main hepatic artery in the hepatoduodenal ligament and porta hepatis may mimic a dilated biliary duct on grayscale imaging. However, color Doppler imaging shows color flow in the enlarged tortuous arteries.[76] Spectral Doppler analysis may exhibit spectral broadening in the region of AVM as well as a high-velocity and low-resistance waveform pattern in the feeding arteries. Analysis of the draining vein shows an arterialized flow pattern with pulsations during systole and a lack of respiratory phasicity. Color and power Doppler ultrasound may be also useful for follow-up of patients after therapeutic embolization or in screening for hepatic abnormalities in the relatives of patients known to have HHT.

CASE 10: RENAL ARTERY EMBOLUS

Case 10. A 65-year-old woman presented with acute flank pain and renal failure. She was believed to have an obstructing stone and was sent to interventional radiology for a nephrostomy and possible stent placement. However, color Doppler image revealed no evidence of hydronephrosis (*A*). In addition, no arterial blood flow was shown in the renal sinus or cortex. (*B*) Transverse color Doppler image of the aorta (A) the left main renal artery (*arrows*). Angiogram confirmed occlusion of the left main renal artery (*arrow*) (*C*). (*Reprinted from* Scoutt LM, Taylor KW. The kidney. In: Taylor KJ, Burns PN, Wells PN, editors. Clinical applications of Doppler ultrasound. 2nd edition. New York: Raven Press; 1995. p. 174–5; with permission.)

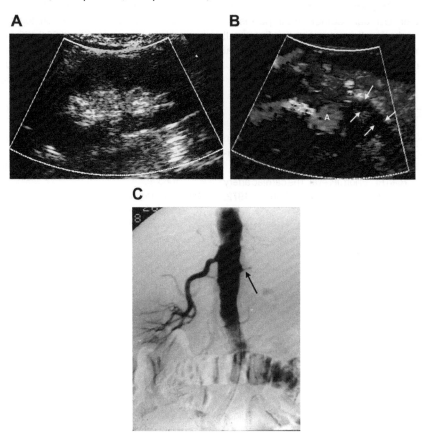

Patients with thromboembolic disease of the renal artery usually present with acute flank pain. Early diagnosis and treatment with anticoagulation, fibrinolytic agents, or embolectomy is crucial to prevent irreversible renal damage.[77–79] Renal artery occlusion can occur because of progression of atherosclerosis from a stenotic lesion to complete occlusion; from an embolic event in the setting of trauma, aortic dissection, or cardiac disease; and as a complication of surgery or percutaneous renal artery angioplasty/stent placement (usually secondary to dissection, disruption or hemorrhage into plaque). The heart is the source of systemic arterial emboli in as many as 94% of patients.[80] The four major causes of systemic emboli are atrial fibrillation, myocardial infarction (postinfarction thrombi typically within ventricular aneurysms), prosthetic valves and rheumatic mitral stenosis.[78] Less common causes of systemic emboli include atrial myxoma, bacterial endocarditis, and atheromatous material from aneurysm or plaque. Only 2% to 3% of peripheral arterial emboli affect the kidney.[80] However, emboli are the most common cause of segmental renal infarcts in the kidney.

Acute renovascular occlusion is often difficult to diagnose and requires a high degree of clinical suspicion. It should be suspected when acute renal failure develops shortly after aortic or renal artery manipulation, particularly if there are signs of extrarenal thromboembolic events. An increased serum lactate dehydrogenase level can be seen in the setting of renal infarction.

On grayscale imaging, no abnormality may be apparent initially. However, color or power Doppler interrogation will reveal complete absence of flow in the renal cortex and main renal artery. In time, the kidney will shrink in size and the renal cortex will become thin and echogenic. Focal or segmental renal infarcts may be either echogenic or hypoechoic on US.[81] Ultimately, areas of parenchymal necrosis can become cystic. Focal infarcts are usually wedge shaped and well defined, but may appear more rounded with indistinct borders. Power Doppler US can depict focal perfusion defects by clearly visualizing surrounding fine small vessels in the rest of the normally perfused renal parenchyma.[82,83]

REFERENCES

1. Horton KM, Talamini MA, Fishman EK. Median arcuate ligament syndrome: evaluation with CT angiography. Radiographics 2005;25:1177–82.
2. Szilagyi DE, Rian RL, Elliott JP, et al. The cardiac artery compression syndrome: does it exist? Surgery 1972; 72:849–63.
3. Bron KM, Redman HC. Splanchnic artery stenosis and occlusion: incidence, arteriographic and clinical manifestations. Radiology 1969;92:323–8.
4. Harjola PT. A rare obstruction of the coeliac artery. Ann Chir Gynaecol Fenn 1963;52:547–50.
5. Duncan AA. Median arcuate ligament syndrome. Curr Treat Options Cardiovasc Med 2008;10:112–6.
6. Loukas M, Pinyard J, Vaid S, et al. Clinical anatomy of celiac artery compression syndrome: a review. Clin Anat 2007;20:612–7.
7. Dumbar JD, Molnar W, Bemon F, et al. Compression of the celiac trunk and abdominal angina. Am J Roentgenol Radium Ther Nucl Med 1965;45:731–44.
8. Wolfman D, Bluth EI, Sossaman J. Median arcuate ligament syndrome. J Ultrasound Med 2003;22:1377–80.
9. Reilly LM, Armmar AD, Stoney RJ, et al. Late result following operative repair for celiac artery compression syndrome. J Vasc Surg 1985;2:79–81.
10. Hibbard LT. Adnexal torsion. Am J Obstet Gynecol 1985;152:456–61.
11. Moore L, Wilson SR. Ultrasonography in obstetric and gynecologic emergencies. Radiol Clin North Am 1994;32:1005–22.
12. Sommerville M, Grimes DA, Koonings PP, et al. Ovarian neoplasms and risk of adnexal torsion. Am J Obstet Gynecol 1991;164:577–8.
13. Cappell MS, Friedel D. Abdominal pain during pregnancy. Gastroenterol Clin North Am 2003;32:1–58.
14. Lee CH, Raman S, Sivanesaratnam V. Torsion of ovarian tumors: a clinicopathological study. Int J Gynaecol Obstet 1989;28:21–5.
15. Chiou SE, Lev-Toaff AS, Masuda E, et al. Adnexal torsion: new clinical and imaging observations by sonography, computer tomography and magnetic resonance imaging. J Ultrasound Med 2007;26: 289–301.
16. Davis AJ, Feins NR. Subsequent asynchronous torsion of normal adnexa in children. J Pediatr Surg 1990;25:687–9.
17. Nissen ED, Kent RD, Nissen SE, et al. Unilateral tuboovarian autoamputation. J Reprod Med 1977;19: 151–3.
18. Andreotti RF, Shadinger LL, Fleischer AC. The sonographic diagnosis of ovarian torsion: pearls and pitfalls. Ultrasound Clin 2007;2:155–66.
19. Anders JF, Powell EC. Urgency of evaluation and outcome of acute ovarian torsion in pediatric patients. Arch Pediatr Adolesc Med 2005;159:532–5.
20. Warner MA, Fleischer AC, Edell SL, et al. Uterine adnexal torsion: sonographic findings. Radiology 1985;154:773–5.
21. Albayram F, Hamper UM. Ovarian and adnexal torsion: spectrum of sonographic findings with pathologic correlation. J Ultrasound Med 2001;20: 1083–9.
22. Vijayaraghavan SB. Sonographic whirlpool sign in ovarian torsion. J Ultrasound Med 2004;23:1643–9.
23. Fleischer AC, Stein SM, Cullinan JA, et al. Color Doppler sonography of adnexal torsion. J Ultrasound Med 1995;14:523–8.
24. Lee EJ, Kwon HC, Joo HJ, et al. Diagnosis of ovarian torsion with color Doppler sonography: depiction of twisted vascular pedicle. J Ultrasound Med 1998; 17:83–9.
25. Tepper R, Zelel Y, Goldberg S, et al. Diagnostic value of transvaginal color Doppler flow in ovarian torsion. Eur J Obstet Gynecol Reprod Biol 1996;68: 115–8.
26. Rollino C, Garofalo G, Roccetello D, et al. Color-coded Doppler sonography in monitoring native kidney biopsies. Nephrol Dial Transplant 1994;9:1260–3.
27. Tung KT, Downes MO, O'Donnell PJ. Renal biopsy in diffuse renal disease: experience with a 14-gauge automatic biopsy gun. Clin Radiol 1992;46: 111–3.
28. Hubsch PJ, Mostbeck G, Barton P, et al. Evaluation of arteriovenous fistulae and pseudo aneurysm in renal allograft following percutaneous needle biopsy. J Ultrasound 1990;9:95–100.
29. Renowden SA, Blethyn J, Cochlin DL. Duplex and color flow sonography in diagnosis of post biopsy arteriovenous fistulae in the transplant kidney. Clin Radiol 1992;45:233–7.
30. Harrison KL, Nghiem HV, Coldwell DM, et al. Renal dysfunction due to an arteriovenous fistula in a transplant patient. J Am Soc Nephrol 1994;5:1300–6.
31. Diaz-Buxo JA, Donadia JV. Complications of percutaneous renal biopsy: an analysis of 1,000 consecutive biopsies. Clin Nephrol 1975;4:223–7.
32. Baquero A, Morris MC, Cope C, et al. Selective embolization of vascular complication following

renal biopsy of the transplant kidney. Transplant Proc 1985;17:1751–2.

33. Hubsch P, Schurawitzki H, Traindl O, et al. Renal allograft arteriovenous fistula due to needle biopsy with late onset of symptoms: diagnosis and treatment. Nephron 1991;59:482–5.

34. Pall AA, Reid AW, Marjorie EM, et al. Renal artery aneurysm six years after percutaneous renal biopsy: successful treatment by embolization. Nephrol Dial Transplant 1992;7:883.

35. Alcazar R, de la Torre M, Peces R. Symptomatic arteriovenous fistula detected 25 years after percutaneous renal biopsy. Nephrol Dial Transplant 1996;11: 1346–8.

36. Smith GH, Remmers AR, Dickey BM, et al. Intrarenal arteriovenous fistula and systolic hypertension following percutaneous renal biopsy: report of a case. Nephron 1968;5:24–30.

37. Goldman ML, Fellner SK, Parrott TS. Transcatheter embolization of renal arteriovenous fistula. Urology 1975;6:386–8.

38. Wolfe JN, Evans WA. Gas in the portal veins of the liver in infants: a roentgenographic demonstration with postmortem anatomical correlation. Am J Roentgenol Radium Ther Nucl Med 1955;74:486–8.

39. Faberman RS, Mayo-Smith WW. Outcome of 17 patients with portal venous gas detected by CT. AJR Am J Roentgenol 1997;169:1535–8.

40. Wiesner W, Mortele KJ, Glickman JN, et al. Pneumatosis intestinalis and portomesenteric venous gas in intestinal ischemia: correlation of CT findings with severity of ischemia and clinical outcome. AJR Am J Roentgenol 2001;177:1319–23.

41. See C, Elliott D. Images in clinical medicine: pneumatosis intestinalis and portal venous gas. N Engl J Med 2004;350:e3.

42. Peloponissios N, Halkic N, Pugnale M, et al. Hepatic portal gas in adults: review of the literature and presentation of a consecutive series of 11 Cases. Arch Surg 2003;138:1367–70.

43. Ruíz DS, de Perrot T, Majno PE. A case of portal venous gas secondary to acute appendicitis detected on gray scale sonography but not computed tomography. J Ultrasound Med 2005;24:383–6.

44. Liebman PR, Patten MT, Manny J, et al. Hepatic portal venous gas in adults: etiology, pathophysiology, and clinical significance. Ann Surg 1978;187:281–7.

45. Lafortune M, Trinh BC, Burns PN, et al. Air in the portal vein: sonographic and Doppler manifestations. Radiology 1991;180:667–70.

46. Nelson AL, Millington TM, Sahani D, et al. Hepatic portal venous gas: the ABCs of management. Arch Surg 2009;144:575–81.

47. Oktar SO, Karaosmanoglu D, Yucel C, et al. Portomesenteric venous gas: imaging findings with an emphasis on sonography. J Ultrasound Med 2006; 25:1051–8.

48. Pan HB, Huang JS, Yang TL, et al. Hepatic portal venous gas in ultrasonogram–benign or noxious. Ultrasound Med Biol 2007;33:1179–83.

49. Ha JF, Phillips M, Faulkner K. Splenic artery aneurysm rupture in pregnancy. Eur J Obstet Gynecol Reprod Biol 2009;146:133–7.

50. Stanley JC, Wakefield TW, Graham LM, et al. Clinical importance and management of splanchnic artery aneurysms. J Vasc Surg 1986;3:836–40.

51. Brockman RL. Aneurysm of splenic artery. Br J Surg 1930;17:692–3.

52. Jack S, Hammond R, James D. Diagnosis and treatment of ruptured splenic artery aneurysm in pregnancy. J Obstet Gynaecol 1997;18:86–7.

53. Sele-Ojeme D, Welch C. Review: spontaneous rupture of splenic artery aneurysm in pregnancy. Eur J Obstet Gynecol Reprod Biol 2003;109: 124–7.

54. Lang W, Strobel D, Beinder E, et al. Surgery of a splenic artery aneurysm during pregnancy. Eur J Obstet Gynecol Reprod Biol 2002;102:215–6.

55. Holdsworth R, Gunn A. Ruptured splenic artery aneurysm in pregnancy. A review. Br J Obstet Gynaecol 1992;99:595–7.

56. Taylor DC, Kettler MD, Moneta GL, et al. Duplex ultrasound scanning in the diagnosis of renal artery stenosis: a prospective evaluation. J Vasc Surg 1988;7:363–9.

57. Kohler TR, Zierler RE, Martin RL, et al. Noninvasive diagnosis of renal artery stenosis by ultrasonic duplex scanning. J Vasc Surg 1986;4:450–6.

58. Strandness DE. Duplex imaging for the detection of renal artery stenosis. Am J Kidney Dis 1994;24: 674–8.

59. Stavros AT, Parker SH, Yakes WF, et al. Segmental stenosis of the renal artery: pattern recognition of tardus and parvus abnormalities with duplex sonography. Radiology 1992;184:487–92.

60. Soares GL, Murphy TP, Singha MS, et al. Renal artery duplex ultrasonography as a screening and surveillance tool to detect renal artery stenosis. A comparison with current reference standard imaging. J Ultrasound Med 2006;25:293–8.

61. Jones RM, Hardy KJ. The hepatic artery: a reminder of surgical anatomy. J R Coll Surg Edinb 2001;46: 168–70.

62. Winter TC, Nghiem HV, Freeny PC, et al. Hepatic arterial anatomy: demonstration of normal supply and vascular variants with three-dimensional CT angiography. Radiographics 1995;15:771–80.

63. Michels NA. Newer anatomy of the liver and its variant blood supply and collateral circulation. Am J Surg 1966;112:337–47.

64. Sahani D, Mehta A, Blake M, et al. Preoperative hepatic vascular evaluation with CT and MR Angiography: implications for surgery. Radiographics 2004; 24:1367–80.

65. Stockx L, Raat H, Caerts B, et al. Transcatheter embolization of hepatic arteriovenous fistulas in Rendu-Osler-Weber disease: a case report and review of the literature. Eur Radiol 1999;9:1434–7.

66. Peery WH. Clinical spectrum of hereditary hemorrhagic telangiectasia (Osler-Weber-Rendu disease). Am J Med 1987;82:989–97.

67. Bernard G, Mion F, Henry L, et al. Hepatic involvement in hereditary hemorrhagic telangiectasia: clinical, radiological and hemodynamic studies of 11 cases. Gastroenterology 1993;105:482–7.

68. Garcia-Tsao G. Liver involvement in hereditary hemorrhagic telangiectasia. J Hepatol 2007;46: 499–507.

69. Baer JW. Hepatic arterioportal fistula related to a liver biopsy. Gastrointest Radiol 1977;2:297–9.

70. Chou YH, Tiu CM. Duplex Doppler ultrasound demonstration of congenital hepatic arteriovenous fistula. J Med Ultrasound 1994;2(4):195–8.

71. Okuda K, Musha H, Yamasaki T, et al. Angiographic demonstration of intrahepatic arterio-portal anastomosis in hepatocellular carcinoma. Radiology 1977; 122:53–8.

72. Winograd J, Palubinskas AJ. Arterio-portal venous shunting in cavernous hemangioma of the liver. Radiology 1977;122:331–2.

73. Cloogman HM, DiCapo RD. Hereditary hemorrhagic telangiectasia: sonographic findings in the liver. Radiology 1984;150:521–2.

74. Thomas JL, Lymberis ME, Hunt TH. Ultrasonic features of acquired renal arteriovenous fistula. AJR Am J Roentgenol 1979;132:653–5.

75. Abramson SJ, Lack EE, Teele R. Benign vascular tumors of the liver in infants: sonographic appearance. AJR Am J Roentgenol 1982;138:629–32.

76. Berland EL, Lawson TL, Foley WD. Porta hepatis: sonographic discrimination of bile ducts from arteries with pulsed Doppler with new anatomic criteria. AJR Am J Roentgenol 1982;138:833–40.

77. Moyer JD, Rao CN, Widrich WC, et al. Conservative management of renal artery embolus. J Urol 1973; 109:138–43.

78. Lessman RK, Johnson SF, Coburn JW, et al. Renal artery embolism, clinical features and long term follow-up of 17 cases. Ann Intern Med 1978;89:477–82.

79. Scolari F, Ravani P, Gaggi R, et al. The challenge of diagnosing atheroembolic renal disease: clinical features and prognostic factors. Circulation 2007; 116:298–304.

80. Fogarty TJ, Buch WS. The management of embolic and thrombotic arterial occlusion. In: Rutherford RB, editor. Vascular surgery. Philadelphia: Saunders; 1977. p. 423–31.

81. Spies JB, Hricak H, Slemmer TM, et al. Sonographic evaluation of experimental acute renal arterial occlusion in dogs. AJR Am J Roentgenol 1984;142:341–6.

82. Huber S, Steinbach R, Sommer O, et al. Contrast-enhanced power Doppler harmonic imaging-influence on visualization of renal vasculature. Ultrasound Med Biol 2000;26:1109–15.

83. Taylor GA, Ecklund K, Dunning PS. Renal cortical perfusion in rabbits: visualization with color amplitude imaging and an experimental microbubble-based US contrast agent. Radiology 1996;201:125–9.

Index

Note: Page numbers of article titles are in **boldface** type.

A

doi:10.1016/S1556-858X(11)00129-0
1556-858X/11/$ – see front matter © 2011 Elsevier Inc. All rights reserved.

ultrasound.theclinics.com

Printed and bound by CPI Group (UK) Ltd, Croydon, CR0 4YY

03/10/2024

01040350-0007